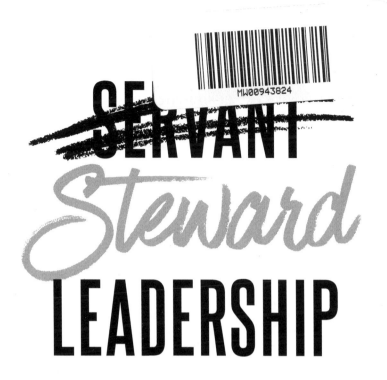

~~SERVANT~~ *Steward* LEADERSHIP

BECOMING A MORE EFFECTIVE LEADER BY BREAKING THE CYCLE OF BEING A HOSTAGE TO YOUR MISSION

DR. KURT PERKINS DC, CCWP

~~SERVANT~~ *Steward* LEADERSHIP

BECOMING A MORE EFFECTIVE LEADER
BY BREAKING THE CYCLE OF BEING
A HOSTAGE TO YOUR MISSION

DR. KURT PERKINS DC, CCWP

KFR
COMMUNICATIONS

First Printing, March 2016

Steward Leadership: Becoming a more effective leader by breaking the cycle of being a hostage to your mission

Copyright © 2016 by Dr. Kurt Perkins DC CCWP

Published in the United States by KFR Communications
www.kfrcommunications.com

Printed in the United States of America

ISBN
Softcover: 978-1519780270

Dedication

To the Women Who Married a Perkins Man.

We are natural workaholics. We love to put our heads down, work, and serve our greater calling in life. It's both a blessing and a curse. Please use this book as a reference guide to create the next generation of the Perkins clan to make sure their servant leadership work doesn't lead to a hostage situation.

Contents

About the Author

I look at creating health, especially as a leader, as a way to worship Him and honor His creation.

Dr. Kurt Perkins, DC CCWP, views health and leadership from a perspective typically contradictory to mainstream outlets.

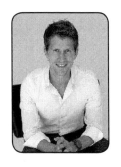

Being the son of a preacher man and a nurse gives him a perspective that can help church leaders be more effective in their missions by taking care of themselves. In short, *find rest before rest finds you.*

Dr. Kurt resides in Colorado Springs, Colorado with his wife Lindsay and three sons, Kalin, Lukas, and Cobi.

Preface

Steadership, Lewardship, you get the point. There's no cool way to combine these words.

I wrote this book because it's time for Christian *leaders* to be *steward* role models. And I'm not singling out the pastors. If you are a mom or dad raising a child in a Christian home, a teacher in a Christian school, or a Christian business owner with employees, than you are a Christian steward and leader with a flock. If you want your flock to follow you, they have to know you can set and keep the pace.

I'm a stewardship, leadership, and health junkie. I'm in a constant state of continually learning. The three can't be separated. There's no greater determining factor on the effectiveness and longevity of a leader than his health. Health isn't just the physical body. There's a physical, chemical, emotional, spiritual, and social aspect to being an effective leader.

The servant leadership problem

I'm of the generation where anytime I listen or read about leadership, the overwhelming theme comes back to the almighty tag line of "servant leadership."

I love the concept of servant leadership and I feel too many leaders have taken that servant aspect into early graves. Push, push, push, until you can't push anymore. Servant leadership has become a hostage situation.

Instead of being synonymous with strength, wisdom, endurance, steadfastness, and sustained energy, leadership has become synonymous with fatigue, burn out, distractions, and illness.

Maybe I'm a little jaded. Maybe I'm a little sensitive to these issues. Let me give you a bit about my background so you know where I'm coming from.

Who's responsible?

I grew up a PK (Pastor's Kid), the youngest of three. My siblings are nine and seven years older. For forty-three years my dad led small and older congregations; no more than fifty people and 65% of those older than sixty. Once my siblings went off to college, I *was* the youth group.

My mom was a nurse. When we had a cough, sniffle, or sneeze, she knew what to observe and what to do.

Being the youngest in a church without much of a voice, I observed people, too. I watched them like crazy on Sunday mornings, Sunday evenings, and Wednesday nights. My overwhelming memory is that a lot of sick people were asking for prayers from each other and for God's help in overcoming their health issues.

I also noticed these people getting sicker and sicker with one, two, or several of the same chronic illnesses that drive 80% of healthcare spending. You know the list: heart disease, cancer, obesity, diabetes, dementias, arthritis, and more.

These were good, faithful people. They didn't miss services. They attended regional camp meetings. They volunteered for anything and everything. They welcomed any visitor to the church with open arms and a seat next to them at the potluck dinner.

They were servants to a higher calling and mission of spreading the Gospel, love, and truth of Jesus Christ. As they got sicker and passed away, so did their mission because there was no younger congregation to pick up their work.

I didn't want their illnesses, and I wondered why God wasn't healing these great, caring, and loving people. Was God missing or was there an action of faith missing?

Being an observer, analytical by nature, and raised in a home where work ethic is king, as an adult I looked to the book of James for a possible answer. And here is what I found in James 2:14-26 English Standard Version (ESV):

Faith Without Works Is Dead

14What good is it, my brothers, if someone says he has faith but does not have works? Can that faith save him? 15If a brother or sister is poorly clothed and lacking in daily food, 16and one of you says to them, "Go in peace, be warmed and filled," without giving them the things needed for the body, what good is that? 17So also faith by itself, if it does not have works, is dead.

18But someone will say, "You have faith and I have works." Show me your faith apart from your works, and I will show you my faith by my works. 19You believe that God is one; you do well. Even the demons believe—and shudder! 20Do you want to be shown, you foolish person, that faith apart from works is useless?

21Was not Abraham our father justified by works when he offered up his son Isaac on the altar? 22You see that faith was active along with his works, and faith was completed by his works; 23and the Scripture was fulfilled that says, "Abraham believed God, and it was counted to him as righteousness"—and he was called a friend of God.

24You see that a person is justified by works and not by

faith alone. ²⁵And in the same way was not also Rahab the prostitute justified by works when she received the messengers and sent them out by another way? ²⁶For as the body apart from the spirit is dead, so also faith apart from works is dead.

Verse 26 sums it up best. If the body is apart from the spirit, then the body is dead. The body is a temporary gift, created in God's likeness, and to be used as a vessel to carry out Christ's great commission. When we don't live healthy, then we are failing as leaders because we are wearing out and destroying what is on loan from God.

Remember, you are a leader, no matter your formal title. As Christians, I'm challenging us all to balance our servant leadership with *Steward Leadership.*

Although we are gaining traction on becoming better stewards of God's resources like our finances and time, we are only as capable as our bodies allow. The number one way to limit our time and financial impact on expanding God's Kingdom is by being poor stewards of our bodies.

Becoming a healthy steward

Stewardship is a combination of beliefs, behaviors, and actions. Behaviors are dictated by beliefs. If you want to know what someone believes, just observe their behaviors and actions. For example, I'm sure you have parishioners who say they don't have money to tithe, yet they drive to church in new and expensive suvs. They also say they don't have time to read their Bibles, yet you see them update their Facebook status every five minutes or brag about binge-watching a favorite tv series.

To be good stewards of our God-given resources, we have to dive deep into why we believe, behave, and act as we do or don't do; to consciously improve; and to be able to see progress so that we're motivated to keep improving. By reading this book, you can begin your own deep dive.

What you'll find in this book

Through this short book, I'll unpack and address aspects of life where you can actually be more productive in your mission by consciously stewarding your health.

In Part I, we'll unpack and learn how to align the 4 Ps of steward leadership; it's a pyramid of philosophy, purpose, psychology, and procedures.

In Part II, we'll tackle some leadership culture practices that directly affect your health and drive your servant leadership into a cycle of hostage negotiations.

And in Part III, you'll learn how to start regaining your health by crafting your own *7-Day Jump Start to Health* program.

From the beginning to the end of this book, I strive to provide you tools, techniques, and strategies you can use to start your physical stewardship journey. So let's get started!

Dr. Kurt Perkins, DC CCWP

www.morehealthlesshealthcare.com

P.S. To find out more about my journey to stewardship health, see the Afterword in this book.

Procedures

Psychology

Purpose

Philosophy

PART I

THE STEWARD LEADERSHIP PYRAMID

You've seen this with new believers. They're excited and on fire about accepting Jesus Christ as their Lord and Savior. Now they want to know exactly what to *do* to keep the fire going.

But here's the thing: God made us human *beings*, not human *doings*. We can only do something for so long before we burn out, even if that something is great for us. When James said that faith without action is dead, he also meant that when our actions die off, so does our faith. So how can you be sure you're fueling your faith with your actions and vice-versa? By aligning the 4 Ps of your steward leadership pyramid.

To paraphrase Ayn Rand, when your Ps don't align, then you'll have contradictions that lead to destruction in propor-

1

tion to your contradictions. As a steward leader, you don't want contradictions.

The flow is the secret

To have success with leadership, health, finances, relationships, or any endeavor you *have* to align your 4 Ps in a bottom-up flow. For examples of why bottom-up is crucial, look to the New Year's resolutions we keep or don't keep.

Chris vows, "I'm going to the gym and exercise at 5 a.m. because I should be healthier," but Chris hates the gym, hates 5 a.m., has a muddy *why*, and no one else except Chris who might benefit.

Contrast that with Pat who vows, "I'm a parent who wants to feed my family. The healthiest food is the food I grow, and I need a stronger back to do it. I'll do exercises to strengthen my back."

Of the two, who is more likely to change their behavior for the long-term? As explained in the next four chapters, it's the one who has their 4 Ps aligned, bottom-up.

Imagine if you turned the pyramid upside-down and onto its point. This would not be stable. Even if you had the most sophisticated dreidel to balance it, eventually it tips over. Keep the flow running upward from the base of the pyramid to the top. You'll be far less likely to tip over and, if you do, you'll find it easier to recalibrate.

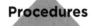

Procedures

Psychology

Purpose

Philosophy
What's my steward leadership role?
Metaphisics

CHAPTER 1

PHILOSOPHY IS A REALITY ROLE

Marcus Aurelius—the last of the five good Roman emperors and one of the most important Stoic philosophers—said:

What then may guide a man? One thing and this only; philosophy.

But this consists in keeping the guardian spirit within a man free from violence and unharmed.

Superior to pains and pleasures, doing nothing without purpose, though yet falsely or with hypocrisy. Not feeling the need of another man's doing or not doing anything.

Moreover, accepting all that happens and all that is allotted as coming from the source wherever it is from whence he himself came.

Aurelius answered the philosophical question, "What does this mean to me?" For Christian leaders, the question is "What's my role in this game of stewardship?"

You're in a leadership role, and times will get tough. It's not a matter of if, but when. Knowing your philosophy helps guide you when times get tough. You have a philosophy whether you consciously formulated it or unconsciously absorbed it. Your philosophy is vital to your leadership effectiveness, especially when making sure you're healthy enough to keep up with leadership demands.

To really dive into how to uncover your philosophy I use the five branches described by Ayn Rand: metaphysics, epistemology, ethics, politics, and aesthetics. I know it's a little ironic since Ayn Rand—in addition to being a philosopher—was an atheist, but the way she breaks down philosophy makes it easier to understand why we act and think differently than others.

Let's get metaphysical

Before you think I'm getting new agey, stay with me on this. Metaphysics gets a bad reputation in the Christian world because it connotes mysticism. But mysticism is just a form of metaphysics. As a Christian, you practice metaphysics more than anyone you know. Your ethical, political, and artistic values are grounded in your metaphysical view.

The fact that you read a Bible is based on your metaphysical view of life and your time on this planet. Whether you tithe is based on your metaphysical view. Even your health outcomes are based on your metaphysical view.

In other words, metaphysics is merely your view of the nature of reality, and this is where arguments between creationists and evolutionists hit the fan. The reality for Christians is that we were created in God's image. The reality for evolutionists is that "we morphed from a primordial goo." And our different views of reality trigger heated debates that often escalate into ethical and political arguments.

Instead of lovingly disagreeing, you, the Christian, want to pummel their heads into the sand. (They will know we are Christians by our love?)

Here's what you and non-Christians have in common: your metaphysical view will drive the other parts of your philosophy—your epistemological, ethical, political, and aesthetic views—and that combination will set the stage for the other parts of your stewardship pyramid: your purpose, psychology, and procedures.

Our daily lives are filled with playbooks of opposing metaphysical views: race relations; the type of reporting that Fox News does in comparison to msnbc; you arguing with your toddler, your teen, or your neighbor.

Though it's easy to see how the metaphysical views of others play out, it may not be easy to truly know what your own views are. So before you make your next political decision, ethical or moral argument, or even artistic expression, I recommend that you really dig into yours. Here's mine:

My metaphysical view is that I am a child of God, created in His image, and given the duty to be a good steward of His resources since my life is only temporary. Humans are predisposed for health, not sickness. When health is not achieved, I am responsible for improving it, even when poor health is not my fault. I am not a victim. Health happens when my faith and my actions meet.

You and other Christians are living in a society led to believe that life is random chance. A society that believes life is random chance is going to believe that is illness is random chance.

As a result, your flock is filled with people who believe their illnesses are due to bad bugs, bad genes, and other types of bad luck. Their doctor tells them "There is nothing more we can do," and it's actually true. There are other options, just not in that doctor's toolbox because a doctor can't give a drug or do surgery to correct a deficiency—not for nutrients, not for movement, and not for relationships.

So you, the Christian leader, are looked upon for comfort and solace and prayer to fix their health problems. You're not equipped to help them in the action department, just the faith department. Just like I'm not equipped to handle them in the faith department, just the action department. But if the church is going to make a difference today, if it's going to attract new believers, dare I say be sexy to the community, then the leaders within the church must have what the lost want but don't have.

What do the lost want? They want what your followers want but don't have either: health that feeds them sustained energy to impact His Kingdom.

YOUR METAPHYSICAL CALL TO ACTION. WHAT DO YOU BELIEVE ABOUT THE WORLD AND YOUR HEALTH?

How now epistemology?

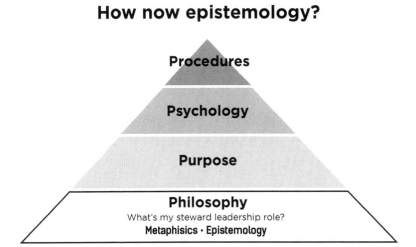

Procedures

Psychology

Purpose

Philosophy
What's my steward leadership role?
Metaphisics · Epistemology

If metaphysics is our nature of reality (what we know), then epistemology answers, "How do we know?" Again, this "proof" is going to create debate. If you're talking with an evolutionist, they won't subscribe to the idea that the Bible is the truth. If you're talking with a Muslim, they have a different set of "truth" texts.

As Christians, we base our faith on our belief that the Bible is God's word and the people who wrote it were God inspired. If our metaphysical view is that we are children of God, created in His image and given the duty to be good stewards of His resources, then how do we know? Because the scriptures tells us so. Genesis 1:27 says (depending on translation):

> *So God created mankind in His own image, in the image of God he created them; male and female he created them.*

Starting with Adam, the scriptures also tell us we're here as temporary stewards of His belongings, and this includes our bodies. We see this in Genesis 2:19:

> *Now out of the ground the Lord God had formed every beast of the field and every bird of the heavens and brought them to the man to see what he would call them. And whatever the man called every living creature, that was its name.*

Talk about instant, on-the-job training for being a steward of God's gifts! That's some serious trust, and if that's you in the Garden of Eden, you don't want to screw it up. You want to make God proud.

How do we know that this life is temporary and that God expects us to be stewards of our bodies while we are here? For one reason, it's blindingly obvious that we're all going to die at some point. If that weren't the case then Adam and Eve would still be around. For another reason, God is pretty clear in Genesis 3:19 about His plan:

> *By the sweat of your brow you will eat your food until you return to the ground, since from it you were taken; for dust you are and to dust you will return.*

There you go, God's plan for health—stewardship of our bodies—was born. You will move well (sweat of your brow) and you will eat well (eat your food). Health is really that simple. A mentor of mine, Dr. James Chestnut, coined the phrase that sums it up: "Eat Well, Move Well, Think Well."

Other ways to argue an epistemological view are via experience, deductive logic, and statistics. I'll be scattering a bit of all three throughout the book.

What we know about cleanliness and pot roasts

This next part illustrates why it's so important for us to *know how we know*. Is our knowledge consciously formulated or subconsciously absorbed?

All the clean ones are in labs. I had a college professor who always said, "Cleanliness is Godliness." We were lab rats and he wanted the lab clean. It was a small, Christian, liberal arts college so he played the Bible card on us until a classmate spoke up and said, "You know that's not in the Bible, right?"

Pot roasts are mysteries. Before putting the pot roast in the pan, the newly wed wife cut off both ends of the roast. Puzzled, her husband asked, "Why did you do that to perfectly good meat?"

"I don't know," she replied, "that's how my mom always made pot roast."

Alarmed, the young man said, "No way, my mom *never* cut off the ends."

Recognizing that this could escalate into a meaningless argument, they called the wife's mom and asked why she cut off the ends of the roast before placing it in the pan. Mom's reply? "That's how your grandmother always did it."

So they called the wife's grandmother. "Grandma, when you make a pot roast, why do you always cut off the ends before putting it in the pan?"

The grandmother had a sensible (for her) answer: "Because my pan is too small. The cut of meat is always too big for the pan so I cut off the ends to make it fit."

How do you know what you know of health?

Once you uncover your metaphysical view, dissect where you got that information. Is your metaphysical view based on a consciously formulated postulate? Or is it a smorgasbord of subconscious absorption of your surroundings?

Our greatest influencers are our parents, teachers, and preachers. Within the health realm, be aware of the massive influence from the pharmaceutical industry and doctors. There are a lot of incentives for them to get you to believe that sickness is normal.

YOUR EPISTEMOLOGICAL CALL TO ACTION. WHAT IS YOUR PROOF SOLIDIFYING YOUR BELIEFS ABOUT HEALTH? ARE YOU OPEN TO QUESTIONING OR VERIFYING YOUR BELIEFS?

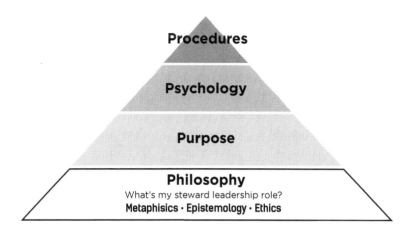

Ethics are not secret codes

Ethics is the branch of philosophy that deals with the nature and purpose of human behavior. When you think of a moral code or a code of values that guides your decisions and actions, then that's ethics.

To be valid, a moral code must address the long-range needs of humans, hold human life as its highest value, and the code must be based on a system of noncontradictory, reliable principles. The Ten Commandments are perhaps the most well-known code of ethics (moral code) ever written. In addition to don't kill, don't cheat, and don't steal, the code includes egoism and altruism commandments.

Egoism is your moral obligation to your own self wellbeing. Altruism is your moral obligation to serve some entity other than yourself at the sacrifice of your own welfare. Extremes in egoism or altruism aren't beneficial to being a long term, effective leader. In fact, servant leadership becomes a hostage situation when church leaders take their mission too far, destroying their own health and then leaving the people they should be serving most (their families) high and dry.

Altruism versus egoism is where we often see arguments about our responsibilities for taking care of our fellow humans. In terms of leadership, I suggest that steward leadership (egoism) should take precedence over servant leadership (altruism) because the former will foster health and keep the latter from turning into a hostage situation.

Far too often, I've seen the servant leader become the overly-altruistic leader and literally destroy their health. In spite of their noble and amazing mission, they don't leave enough in their tank to serve their own families. Or perhaps even worse, they destroy their health to a point where no amount of service *to* them from others will help them continue their mission.

The leader becomes the focal point instead of their mission, sabotaging the original purpose and intent of the venture. There has to be a balance between egoism (taking care of yourself) and altruism (taking care of others).

Ignoring one's health is an ethical issue. Since human life is the highest moral value, doing things (or not doing things) to protect and preserve a human life (your health) is a contradiction in our Christian ethical code.

Let me be clear: your level of health won't be a determining factor in your salvation. It's not a salvation issue. It's an obedience issue. It's where faith meets action.

YOUR ETHICAL CALL TO ACTION. IS YOUR HEALTH STRATEGY TRULY ETHICAL AND LONG-LIVED, OR IS IT IMBALANCED AND SHORT TERM?

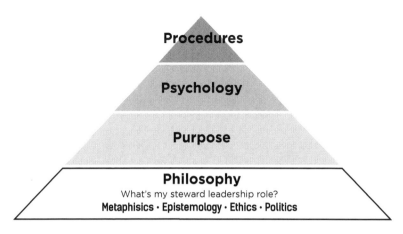

Politics made easy

Politics is taking what applies to an ethical setting to a social setting. In other words, it takes what is good for an individual and tries to apply that to everyone.

If killing a baby is harmful for one baby then it will be harmful for all babies. This is why many Christians take a stance against abortion. Our moral code, the Ten Commandments, says do not murder.

The entire nervous system, the one system that organizes and coordinates *every* function in the body is formed by eight weeks postconception. At this time, all systems of the body are a go.

But when *life* begins goes back to a person's metaphysical and epistemological views. What's the nature of reality? Does life begin at conception or does life happen at birth? How do I know?

You can see why so many political debates happen over this one issue alone.

I support the causes that keep human life as its standard of value, and because I know my true metaphysical and epistemological views, then it's easy for me to take a political stance. If the issue contradicts my metaphysical and epistemological view, then I oppose it. If it doesn't matter either way to me, I flip a coin.

Just to be clear, I oppose government run healthcare. Healthcare does *not* create health; instead it focuses on a minimum standard of health defined by the presence or absence of symptoms. If you have enough symptoms, then you get treatment until the symptoms go away. Not enough symptoms? Sorry, you're not sick enough, or you're now well enough to take off government care. That makes government run healthcare a contradiction for those seeking true health. The only viable solution to creating true health is through steward leadership.

Just look at the past forty years. In the late 70s, heart disease and obesity were rising, and the government was pressuring the medical industry to take action. So the medical industry responded by declaring war on fat and cholesterol.

And what has happened? A contradiction. Americans have *lower* cholesterol rates now than in the 70s, but *higher* rates of heart disease and obesity. And to deal with those and other health problems, we now have government-imposed "healthcare" and even more incentives to keep people sick.

The same situation happened with the flu shot. Prior to 1980, only about 15-20% of people aged 65 and up got a yearly flu shot. By 2001, over 60% of that same population was getting a yearly flu shot. What happened to flu-associated deaths? Oh, they increased. To force people to get a flu shot based on dogma and "that's the way we have always done it" contradicts my metaphysical and epistemological views, so I will vote against it.

I do support free market HSA type insurance plans or medical sharing plans where people can choose what to do with their healthcare money and reserve using insurance for its original intended purpose...emergencies.

In fact, today's insurance is a prime example of our broken healthcare system; we are now treating chronic conditions with emergency money and in emergency settings. And that contradicts the purpose of insurance.

If your house is on fire, you want the fire department. They may break some windows, bust a couple doors, and soak a couple walls but they saved your house.

Once the fire is out, you don't call the fire department to rebuild it. You call contractors, painters, carpenters, and dry wallers because they have the right tools. The fire department has the wrong tools. You wouldn't call the carpenter to try and put a fire out with a hammer and nails.

Yet, our government-sponsored healthcare system supports emergency interventions for all health conditions. Our healthcare system is saturated with 80% of the time and money being spent to treat chronic conditions (poor stewardship of illness) with emergency interventions.

Regrettably, in the servant leader's world of serve, serve, serve, many don't do anything. They ignore their chronic conditions. They let the house burn down. They are too spent to call 911. Perhaps that servant leader expects to be bailed out by his faithful flock; sadly, it doesn't work that way much of the time.

Sure, there are feel good stories of communities coming together to help, but did this change the servant leader's heart and behavior to never again be a burden to his flock; or is he going to repeat his cycle of exhaustion, fatigue, and illness? Wayne Muller puts it best:

> *If we do not allow for the rhythm of rest in our overly busy lives, illness becomes our Sabbath—our pneumonia, our cancer, our heart attack, our accidents create Sabbath for us.*

At the time of this writing, my dad has Alzheimer's and his colleagues of more than forty years won't visit him because they feel uncomfortable. As a servant leader, my dad poured himself into their lives, and where are those people now? I know his reward is in Heaven but I also know he wanted to mentor up-and-coming pastors. Now all he can do is tell a story about how he went to the zoo in the third grade and his dad commenting that his son went to the zoo but a monkey came back instead...over and over again.

So know this: to *not* consciously take care of yourself is an ethical and moral dilemma in your life as a leader. I don't want you miserable healthy. I want you healthy because it's a sign of obedience to God's calling on taking care of what He owns and has asked you to shepherd.

If someone lends you some tools, they know you are going to use them. They will incur some wear and tear and not be perfect but you wouldn't leave them out in the rain, run them over with your car, or get paint all over them. You will return the tools to your friend in the best possible condition. This is how you should view and treat your body.

How do you do that? I cover it in the second half of this book, providing guidance on how to get and stay healthy so you really do feel like you were created in God's image.

I don't know about you, but I don't picture God fat, poor postured, constantly sweating, on antidepressants, and starting his day with coffee and donuts. Which leads us to the fifth aspect of philosophy: aesthetics.

YOUR POLITICAL CALL TO ACTION. WHAT POLITICAL VIEWS MIGHT YOU HOLD THAT ARE DISCOURAGING YOUR HEALTH?

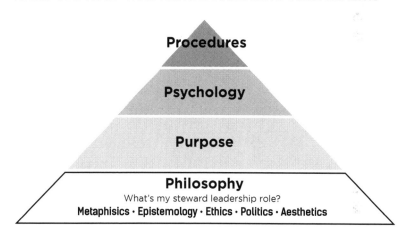

Procedures

Psychology

Purpose

Philosophy
What's my steward leadership role?
Metaphisics · Epistemology · Ethics · Politics · Aesthetics

Aesthetics made obvious

Aesthetics is a man's relationship with beauty. To quote Ayn Rand again:

> *Art is a selective re-creation of reality according to the artist's metaphysical value judgments.*

What are you doing to re-create the reality of your metaphysical view? How are you outwardly expressing your view of the nature of reality?

I took one art history course in college...because I had to. I don't remember a thing about it. It was a lot of memorization of dates and eras when I already had enough to remember with chemistry and biology. But if I were to take that course again, I think I would be more interested in trying to guess the metaphysical view of the artist just based on their work. For example, if the artist always depicts humans in a weak, worn down, decrepit posture, then what does that say about their aesthetic representation of their metaphysical view?

Maybe the art form isn't in sculptures or paintings. Maybe it's in the spoken word. For example, compare someone who is always complaining to the person who is always gracious, kind, and holds their tongue, even when times are tough. You say that's a personality difference? I say, again, that's the aesthetic expression of a metaphysical view.

Even your doctor's recommendations are an aesthetic expression of a metaphysical view. If your doctor puts you on blood pressure medication with no exit strategy or says something to the tune of "when diet and exercise fail," then he's expressing his metaphysical view. You might even be told that you are predisposed to x illness. I say that's crap because it opposes my reality of the nature of health.

When you were designed in the image of the one and only God, the only thing you were predisposed to was unbelievable health. Your DNA is set up to not only survive life but to help life thrive.

Is your outward expression—your aesthetic—one that matches the other aspects of your philosophical view? Do you look at yourself in the mirror and think, "This is the image of God." When your feet hit the floor in the morning and you take those first few steps, do you think, "I feel great, I bet God feels great!"

YOUR AESTHETIC CALL TO ACTION. HOW DO YOU TALK ABOUT YOUR HEALTH? WHEN YOU SEE PICTURES OF YOURSELF, DO YOU SEE A WELL CARED-FOR VESSEL OR A VESSEL IN NEED OF CARE?

Your philosophy action plan

The more you work on your physical health, the more you can carry out your God-given mission. I know it personally because when I'm practicing discipline, then the other aspects of life get better. I'm more diligent with my Bible reading. My relationships with my wife and kids are better. Ultimately, I'm able to serve my patients more effectively and be the example they are looking for.

People in general want to know that their leaders are practicing what they are preaching. This is especially true in the church and one of the biggest criticisms of the church... that it's filled with hypocrites.

But again, to experience God's blessings you have to be intentional. Servant leadership to the point of exhaustion and burnout is not being intentional.

Stewardship leadership to the point that you still have energy to serve your family and be well enough to be served is intentional. Start being intentional by becoming very clear about the first of the 4 Ps: your philosophy. Here's how.

1. Formulate your metaphysical view as a steward from multiple angles. Consider your health, marriage, child rearing, finances, and so on. This isn't a 5-minute exercise. Analyze, pray, journal, and uncover your view of reality. You may uncover beliefs that surprise you.

2. Uncover your epistemological view. Once you uncover your metaphysical view (step 1), dissect where you got your information. Does your metaphysical view appear to be a Christian view but you can't actually support it with scripture (your epistemological view)? Expect to find contradictions. Better to recognize and clear them up now because contradictions eventually lead to destruction.

3. Make sure your ethical view aligns with your metaphysical and epistemological view. How will you behave when the chips are down? Contradictions lead to destruction. The destruction is proportional to the level of contradiction. Choose the one issue that dictates your voting record and political backing. I encourage you to position human life as your highest value.

4. Determine your political views. How do you believe society should behave to align with your ethical view? If there is a candidate who supports all your ideals but is against your highest value, this could be a contradiction you need to clear up.

5. Assess your aesthetics. Do you look, feel, and act like you are an image of God? Would God look at you and say, "that's not really what I had in mind?" If you're preaching how great and powerful God is, yet complaining of chronic health problems, fatigue, and sweating just to walk to the pulpit, then you have work to do. Activate your ego and work towards becoming the outward expression of how it looks, sounds, and feels to be made in God's image.

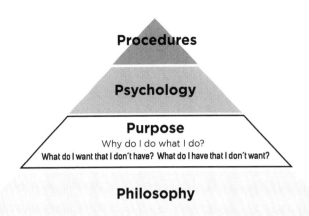

Procedures

Psychology

Purpose
Why do I do what I do?
What do I want that I don't have? What do I have that I don't want?

Philosophy

CHAPTER 2

PURPOSE IS YOUR BIG WHY

Philosophy answers the question, "What's my role in life?" Purpose answers the question, "Why do I do what I do?" or "What do I want that I don't have?"

If you've read any leadership books, then you know that the author almost always hits on the why behind leadership. I want to hit on why you do or don't' do what you can for your health. In my experience, a person's health *why* is the greatest driver that leads them to succeed or fail in caring for themselves.

Anyone's *why* can be broken down into either gaining something you want but don't have or into getting rid of something you have but don't want. The people who fail the most often are the ones trying to get rid of something they have but don't want. Instead of gaining strength, they are trying to get rid of weight. Instead of gaining financial independence, they are trying to get rid of debt. Instead of forming a good habit, they are trying to get rid of a bad habit.

The more you focus on gaining something you want but don't have, the more apt you are to put up with the hard times, overcome roadblocks, push ahead, and stay the course. For me, my health and leadership journey comes down to three main whys: money, vanity, and legacy (all in a good way).

Spend smart

It's not that I won't pay for things. It's that I *hate* paying for stupid things. Every year Fidelity and other investment companies routinely report that retiring couples are going to need roughly $250,000 in savings to pay for healthcare needs. This is on *top* of what Medicare will cover.

With 80% of our healthcare system jammed with chronic conditions, that just tells me that's 80% of the population is making stupid decisions about their health; or that they and their doctors share a metaphysical view of the body as a pile of parts destined to wear out, and disease is due to bad bugs, bad genes, and bad luck.

I believe that most chronic illness is lifestyle illness. And being chronically ill due to circumstances that are truly beyond our control does not lessen our responsibility to take control.

Reading this, you may be getting hot under the collar because you lost a loved one, even someone very young, from a chronic illness that wasn't their fault. Fair enough. But we're not absolved of our stewardship responsibility to do what we can. Consider, for example, what we can and can't do about the money spent on health.

The insurance contradiction

As originally conceived, health insurance was designed to cover *emergency* situations. Not so today. Instead of just emergencies, we're now using health insurance to apply emergency interventions to lifestyle problems.

Here's the contradiction: What other insurance industry besides health insurance allows you to destroy your property and then claim it as a loss and get reimbursed? None.

You can't start a bon fire in your living room because you like the smell and expect your homeowner's insurance to rebuild your house when you burn it down.

You can't call up your auto insurance carrier and expect them to pay for gasoline, tires, and car washes.

We're responsible for being stewards of our homes, autos, and other property we own or borrow, why not our most valuable property of all: our bodies, the property we've borrowed from God?

The more we pay for healthcare interventions, the more disease we have. We don't have a healthcare system, we have a sick care system. And the solution isn't to spend more money and give everyone access to it. The solution is to turn those who are spending into a broken system into investors of their own health, as beings who are fearfully and wonderfully made in the image of God..

So here's a suggestion: Opt for the high deductible HSA plan and start putting money into your health today so can you save $250,000 in healthcare expenses when you retire, if you make it to retirement. My brother didn't.

The politics and money that make us sick

There's a lot of money that goes into industries that aren't as regulated as you might think, such as the chemical and sugar industries, and even the vaccine industry. Let's take a brief look at what it means for our health.

Chem(sick)les

Of the over 80,000 industrial chemicals in use in America today—many of which are banned in other countries—only a small percentage have mandated testing. Also, the mandated testing usually applies only if the chemical is carcinogenic, even though chemicals are more notorious for being *hormone disruptors* than for being carcinogens.

How many in your flock have thyroid, testosterone, or estrogen problems?

Of the many chemicals on the market, the epa has only been successful at banning or removing five: polychlorinated biphenyls, dioxin, hexavalent chromium, asbestos and chlorofluorocarbons. (See http://www.nytimes.com/2013/04/14/sunday-review/think-those-chemicals-have-been-tested.html)

A small study by the Environmental Working Group in

2005 involved taking the cord blood of ten newborns. These babies were minutes old, not even exposed to any outside influence. Blood samples revealed 287 industrial chemicals in their cord blood. Industrial! These are not chemicals God needed to create a fearfully and wonderfully made human.

Of the 287 chemicals, 180 are known cancer causing agents, 217 are toxic to the brain and nervous system, and 208 cause birth defects and/or abnormal development. (See http://www.ewg.org/research/body-burden-pollution-newborns)

Is it surprising, then, that childhood cancer, adhd, autism, anxiety, hormone issues, and allergies to anything and everything are rising?

Patients, parents, doctors, and others want to blame illness and disorders on genetics. But if a disorder is due to genetics, then there should be evidence of the disorder from birth. For example, diseases like Huntington's, sickle cell anemia, and Krabbe disease are evident at or within a few months of birth, and no amount of lifestyle change will improve that gene expression.

Let's be clear: family illness history is not the same as genetic disorder history. Family illness history is lifestyle and behavior history. Using my family history of illness as an example, it's amazing I lived past 20.

Sugar hideouts and vaccine sanctuaries

Here's something you might not know about sugar: on a food label, every item has a percentage of recommended daily allowance...*except* sugar. Now that's a strong lobby.

As for vaccines, it's the only industry where the government has granted sanctuary. If something happens to your child, the government has lifted responsibility from the vaccine manufacturer. Whatever your thoughts about vaccines, when you take away any legal ramifications for an entire industry, don't you think they will cheat a little?

Aligning your money with your purpose

Finding your purpose means answering the question, "What do I want that I don't have?" If you're not healthy now or you want a better shot at staying healthy, you're going to have to question the oxymoron of health insurance, distrust government policy a bit, second-guess your doctor often, and spend your health dollars wisely.

Be vain, very vain

I kind of jest in using the term vanity since it's a subset of pride, one of the seven deadly sins. Pride is excessive belief in one's own abilities, and it interferes with the individual's recognition of the grace of God. Pride—a.k.a. vanity—has been called the sin from which all other sins arise. Thomas Aquinas said of it:

> *The root of pride is found to consist in man not being, in some way, subject to God and His rule.*

What it all comes down to is that I want my wife to look at me when we're 80 and when she does, I want her to do a double take. I want to be the 70 year old at the gym where all the 20-something's are arguing over my real age and no one is guessing over 55.

I want to be the dad challenging my kids with, "Knock it off, don't make me come over there," and being there in a split second and holding my own, even when they are grown adults. I want them to know that our calling to be God's great stewards doesn't end. We are fearfully and wonderfully made and we should show that to the world.

You want to be an effective leader? Be what others want yet don't have. They will follow. I believe your doctor should be the healthiest person you know, otherwise why would you take their health advice? Should the same be true for pastors and leaders of our spiritual health?

Live your legacy

Legacy is my ultimate why. You can create a great legacy in poor health, but I'd rather create mine in good health.

Like President Theodore Roosevelt, I want a great living legacy. He was a sickly, asthmatic child who overcame his health problems by practicing an intentionally strenuous lifestyle.

In addition to good health, I want my legacy to be liquid. Too often our legacy is talked about after we have died. I want my kids and grandkids to look at me when I'm 85 and still want my advice, and to hear about my life experiences, and be open to words of wisdom.

I talk to my mom on the phone every Sunday and in the background you hear someone howling. It's my dad doing crazy noises from his Alzheimer's...at 71. There's no having a conversation about anything meaningful; there's no conversation at all. He comprehends "What do you want to eat for lunch?" and not much else.

Dad was a minister for 43 years. If I ever met someone in public who knew my father, they would always say, "He's the kindest man I've ever known." Now they say their kids are a little weirded out by him, or that he's holding a hand shake way *too long* and *too hard*. Now they won't even visit to see how my mom is doing because they don't want to be around my dad.

Is it my dad's fault that he has Alzheimer's? Maybe. Maybe not. It doesn't matter. But now he is my mom's responsibility. They worked their whole lives, scraped and saved like crazy to put three kids through college, and set themselves up to travel in retirement. Now they're both confined to the house 23 hours per day.

My older brother, Keith, was a superman in my eyes. Nothing could hurt this guy. He rolled cars with only a scratch, knocked out teeth playing sports, went face first into a pricker bush while sledding, and never cried.

Fast forward to adulthood. A young man with a great work ethic, three kids, part owner of an engineering firm, and on fire for God and for creating a great legacy for his family. He almost did, except he lost track of the health part. When there was an immediate goal—like a rafting trip in the Grand Canyon—Keith pursued health. He didn't pursue health as a long-term goal.

At 37, after a three-week business trip, he should have been reuniting with his family. Instead, he was found dead in his hotel room.

Here are his final Facebook updates.

Here's what happened next: Keith made it home in a coffin.

He left a widow, three kids without a dad, and many other sad people. Did he leave a legacy? No doubt. He always said he didn't have many friends, and he was a liar. I spoke at his funeral to a crowd of over 500 people, from all stages of his life, from all parts of the country.

Keith Perkins
August 8, 2009 ·

On my way home Sunday. 27 hours of travel all in 14 clock hours. Gotta love international travel.

Like · Comment · Share

Keith Perkins
August 10, 2009 ·

Didn't quite make it home. Flight cancelled in Newark. What will be next?

Like · Comment · Share

Part of Keith's legacy was his choice in nutrition. As everyone left his funeral, they were handed a can of Mountain Dew and a pack of Reese's Peanut Butter Cups. He often joked that was his breakfast of champions.

Your purpose action plan

I will constantly work to create my own legacy, and to be around so I can watch my kids grow into theirs. Did God use Keith? Absolutely. Was he a leader? Absolutely. Would better stewardship of his body have allowed Keith to be around today to further God's mission?

While I can only speculate about Keith, I can do more for myself. You can, too. Here's how to find your purpose by finding your *why*. Just ask yourself two questions:

1. What is it that you want but don't have that will motivate you to be a better leader and steward of God's Kingdom?

2. To be a better steward of your body, what aspects of health do you want more of?

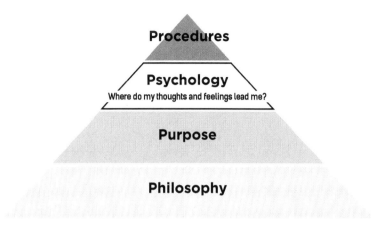

Procedures

Psychology
Where do my thoughts and feelings lead me?

Purpose

Philosophy

CHAPTER 3

PSYCHOLOGY IS YOUR BRAIN ON DOING

In the previous chapters, we covered philosophy and purpose, which together establish your beliefs and form your "compass for being."

In this chapter and the next we'll cover psychology and procedures, which together form your "roadmap for doing."

Sequence is still key

When I introduced the idea of the 4 Ps in Chapter 1, I stressed the importance of aligning your Ps from the bottom-up, from philosophy to purpose to psychology to procedures. The flow is especially crucial if you're trying to change behavior, whether it's your own or the behavior of those you lead.

This is why it's so frustrating to deal with a 3 year old. They have enough mental capacity to understand what you want them to do (procedure) but not enough to understand why you want them to do it (purpose). Psychology does wonders to close the gap.

Toddler psychology

When my oldest son was potty training, we thought it would be easy. At 18 months old he would go into the bathroom to poop (good understanding) either in his diaper or on the floor (not good). For the next two years, the more we forced him to sit on the potty, the more push we had. And not the push of poo going into the water.

One day, we took away all pull-up diapers and told him, we don't care where you poop, you just have to clean it up.

He went into the bathroom, pulled down his pants and popped a squat on the floor, right next to the toilet. No reaction, here's some paper towels, clean it up. He did the best he could at cleaning it up, whined quite a bit about it but that was the last time he ever pooped outside of the potty.

He finally understood *why* we wanted him to poop in the potty. It's gross and stinky to clean up poop. It's much easier to clean and manage in the toilet. His psychology changed about poop and therefore his behaviors.

It's not going to be that easy for you and I. We're bigger

kids who throw bigger tantrums. The process is going to be longer and more painful at times, starting with why changing our behavior is beneficial to ourselves, our families, and our steward leadership roles.

Stewardship and leadership psychology

You may be in a sweet groove with your leadership and really building momentum and influence. Which means you may also be afraid to take time off or step back for fear of losing momentum. I would argue this is the perfect moment to step back and figure out how to build up your own health and disciplines—to change your psychology, if you will—so you can sustain the pace you need to be an effective leader. Don't let poor health turn you into the inmate running the asylum.

Just like I'm challenging a sacred cow of servant leadership, steward leadership is going to be a challenge for you to get your mind around. You will always be in service as a leader. You're just not going to do it to a point of burnout where you ignore and sacrifice the people who should receive your best service.

With psychology, you have to be okay with positive affirmations. You have to verbally state and mentally recognize your personal accomplishments and be proud of your efforts. You may think this is silly stuff but, as Proverbs 4:23 shows, it's biblical:

Above all else, guard your heart, for it is the well-spring of life.

We could take this literally and go on a heart health campaign but in figurative language, whenever someone says they have a broken heart, or "I feel it in my heart," they are verbalizing their emotional experience.

Emotions are a reaction to our circumstances. We choose what emotions to display and share. If you feel proud of your accomplishments, while giving glory to God, you will keep trucking. If you feel unworthy of success or beat yourself up over setbacks, you'll eventually give up.

So guard your heart (your psychology). Be careful what you think and say to yourself. Your psychology is part of your nervous system, and your nervous system is like plastic. The more you repeat something; the more it becomes a default setting.

Be aware and conscious of how you react in different situations. Are you in control of your thoughts and emotions or are you flying off the handle?

There are times to get pissed and act on it. Even Jesus did this. Remember the *Temple as a marketplace* incident (Matthew 21:12-13, Esv)? But he was cool and calm when faced with insults, torture, and false accusations.

Thomas Edison was famous for how he handled stress, and here's an example. One day he received word that his laboratory and factory were on fire. The fire was so ferocious that firemen from eight stations were rushing to the scene.

Instead of panicking, getting angry, and depressed, Edison gathered his wife and kids and headed to the fire, excited to show them the most beautiful flames they would probably ever see. Because of the chemicals used in his lab, the flames were neon yellow and green and estimated to be six-to-seven stories high.

What good would it have been to weep and mourn? Would that have changed the outcome? Would that have stopped the fire? Despite the potential of losing a lifetime's worth of work and progress, Edison embraced the fire for its beauty.

The buildings were supposedly made of fire-proof concrete and so Edison and his investors were only insured for about a third of the damage. Still no negative reaction. He just chalked it up to getting rid of some old rubbish.

In Edison's time, his loss was about $1 million; in 2015 dollars, that's the equivalent of $23 million. Within three weeks of the fire, the factory was partially back up and running. By four weeks the employees were back to work, doing double shifts, and churning out products the world had never seen.

Despite the setback, Edison's venture earned about $10 million in revenue that year. That is the equivalent of $200+ million today. His psychology (not giving up, pushing on) dictated his behaviors.

Edison was already a proven success and winner. In his mind, if he could create it once, he could create it again. Wins build confidence.

The amazing thing is that you, too, have the capacity for Edison-like mind control. This is a skill you can learn. You can choose how you react, you think, and whether you guard your heart. Or as it says in Romans 5:3-4 (paraphrased):

Trials and tribulations...build perseverance, perseverance builds character, and character builds hope.

We're all going to have trials in life. You're going to have leadership trials and health trials. Be thankful for them. Love that you have the trials because you know if you can endure, there's hope for a better outcome in the end.

Hope is a powerful thing. Look how the hopeful people you lead act versus those who feel hopeless. People in the same circumstances, with the same obstacles, will have drastically different outcomes based on their level of hope. Hope creates joy and happiness, and it all stems from our thoughts and feelings, not our behaviors or circumstances.

According to Shawn Achor, author of *How Happiness Fuels Your Success*, only 10% of your level of happiness can be predicted by your external circumstances, like where you live, guaranteed opportunities, and access to wealth. But 90% of your happiness is based on how your brain is processing the world you find yourself in; i.e., how you think about your money, how you think about your position in life, and how you think about your family. In *The Law of Happiness*, author Henry Cloud cites similar statistics.

For example, there are at least two reasons why people who lose everything are often happier than those who merely have setbacks. One reason is optimism, and the other is social connection. Psychologically, they are optimistic that they can eventually improve their situation and—even in chaos—they find meaning and joy in family and friends.

I think one of the hardest struggles that church leaders face is deep, meaningful connections. You lead a lot of people but are essentially isolated. I don't ever remember my dad going out to hang with the guys. Though a leader, he was isolated.

Stewardship isn't just an action; it's a mindset. Your mindset will lead to action, whether good or bad. In fact, your mindset will drive your behavior, even if you don't know what your mindset is. That's because unconscious beliefs will set you in motion.

Do you say being debt free is important, yet just financed the latest and greatest iPhone? Do you say that relationships are key in your family, yet as soon as you get home from work, you're glued to your TV? Do you think that health is very important yet you can't remember the last time you did a pushup or had a glass of water? It's time to assess and maybe change your psychology.

Your psychology action plan

To assess your personal psychology, you need to figure out where your thoughts and feelings are leading you about your health and being responsible for it. Are they leading you towards what you assert you believe and value—as demonstrated by your behavior—or away? Here's how to find out:

1. Track what you do, say, think, and feel for a few days.

2. Affirm or discover your values.

3. Find and resolve incongruences between your psychology and your values.

Congratulate yourself, get to work, or both.

Track what you do, say, think, and feel

The point of this exercise is to become mindful of your mind so that you can work towards recognizing and resolving incongruences.

1. Schedule two to four days to track yourself, making sure you have a split of typical workdays and non-workdays.

2. On each scheduled day, set a timer that alerts you at short, odd intervals—such as every 18 minutes and 57 seconds—for eight hours. (Yes, there are apps for that.)

3. Whenever that timer goes off, jot down what you are doing, saying, thinking, or feeling at that moment.

4. At the end of the day, review each entry. Is it congruent with your philosophy and purpose?

Affirm or discover your values

To affirm your values—or if you don't know your values—do this exercise.

1. Imagine you have a new baby. See your baby, name your baby.

2. You know in 18 years, your child will leave your house and be crowned the new leader of the free world. What characteristics would you want to develop in your child to prepare them to lead the world? Write it down, now. Use this space:

3. Review your list from step 2. You may notice it looks similar to the fruits of the spirit: patience, kindness, slow to anger, love, joy, faithfulness, peace, goodness, gentleness, and self control.

There's no irony in this exercise; no matter your religion, ethnicity, gender, race, or financial status, we humans share many of the same values.

You may be a pastor of a Christian church. You value honesty. So do the terrorists in isis; like you, they don't want to be lied to. You pray for people. They pray for people before they kill them. You're each being congruent with your values based on your philosophy.

Find and resolve your incongruences

So you have your list of mental, verbal, and emotional entries (your psychology) and your list of values. It's time to find and resolve any incongruences.

1. Draw a chart with your entries for your psychology (what you say, think, feel) down the side, and your entries for your values across the top.

2. At the intersection of each entry, enter Yes or No. (It's kind of like the note you passed to your crush in grade school. Do you like me? Yes or No?)

3. Imagine you have a new baby. See your baby, name your baby. Examine your chart. Are all of your thoughts, feelings, words, and actions congruent with your values? If all of your answers are congruent, you're light years ahead of the curve. If not, then be thankful that God gave you the free agency to change.

Congratulate yourself, get to work, or both

When you have all your entries analyzed, pat yourself on the back for all the situations you were congruent. Be proud that you handled yourself in a manner consistent with your values. Be thankful.

For all the entries when you weren't congruent, think of how you could have handled that situation better. I don't mean how you could have handled it perfectly, but just one step better. For example, you value kindness, but when someone cut you off in traffic, you yelled, flipped the bird, and tailgated to retaliate. Well, you've got some work to do. Next time someone cuts you off, instead of flipping the bird, maybe one step better would be to grip the steering wheel tighter so your hand can't come off.

Start now, taking small achievable steps. Build up some psychological wins.

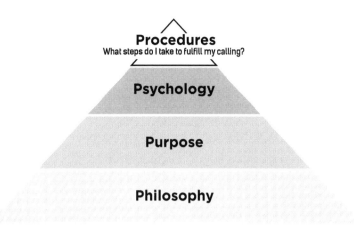

Procedures
What steps do I take to fulfill my calling?

Psychology

Purpose

Philosophy

CHAPTER 4

PROCEDURES ARE DOING YOUR DO

To improve your health and be a better steward of your body so you can lead more effectively, I want you to understand concepts first. If you can get the big idea, the details make a lot more sense and will fall into place better.

With your stewardship action plan, there are a few things I want you to build around: your health tithe, your *one* thing, your first love, your addictions, and the dangers of a particular four-letter word.

Give tithing to your health

The first concept is that you should look at your stewardship plan as a tithe. Tithing isn't just giving 10% of your resources back to the local church. Tithing is about giving 10% of your *first* and *best* resources. Don't get hung up on the 10% part. Get focused on the *first* and *best* part.

Let's say you plan on going for a run after work. You had a long day and felt like you were more of a fire chief putting out fires all day than a leader engaged in developing yourself, team, or tribe.

By the time you get home, you're exhausted. Your spouse made your dinner and you are grateful. Now your belly is full and all you want to do is sit on the couch and catch up on Master Chef.

There's no chance of you going for a run now; it would be like trying to tithe with your last 10%, not your first and best 10%. If you're going to be a good steward of the physical body that God gave you, created in His image, and you desire to give it your best, you're going to have to get used to doing things in the morning, before you put out fires all day.

Not everyone is a morning person. So why do I say the morning? Because mornings are typically when you have the fewest distractions. If someone texts you at 5:30 am., it better be for a good reason.

From a hormone standpoint, mornings will be your biggest natural boost of energy. Cortisol, an adrenal hormone designed to dump sugar into your blood to give you energy, should be the highest in the morning. If you're dragging in the morning that may be a sign you're already into leadership burnout.***

I placed asterisks after that statement because if you're

going to bed at 2 am and expecting to get up at 5:30 am, you're going to be dragging. This is yet another issue for servant leaders that can be solved by going through the 4 Ps.

They get up early to get going on the mission, and come home at night exhausted, with no possible gumption left to work on themselves.

This also applies to stay-at-home parents; they have the most exhausting leadership role in the world. Unless you start the day with your best 10% effort to give back to God, you might not be able to give Him even your last 3% at the end of the day.

When you think about your best 10%, think beyond just exercise. Whatever part of your health that you need to take better stewardship of to be a better leader, do it when you can give your *best* 10%. This could be journaling. This could be drinking water. This could be connecting physically with your spouse. This could be that deep, social connection who wants your friendship and not your leadership.

How many times have you gotten to the end of the day and you, your spouse, or both of you are too tired for some intimate time? You can still kiss each other good night and plan on some sex before dawn. Just saying. Hint, hint Lindsay (my wife).

I'm a morning person. I want to get up and get going. I've never consumed coffee early in the morning to get me going. I'd rather start my day at 4:30 am and give my best eight hours and be done by early afternoon.

The challenge with leadership, in any capacity is that life

happens and we may not always be able to use our best time of day to work on our health stewardship; but we should still keep trying. Put yourself at your best time of day on the calendar and block it out.

How many churches suffer financially because the congregation is trying to give tithe *after* paying their bills and having their fun? Their 10% tithe intention manifested into an actual 2-3% of giving. Your health efforts are no different.

Choose your *one* thing

You can't do everything you want to do with your best 10% of effort. So focus on the one thing that, when you give your best effort, will make all your other efforts easier, even on your last 10% of energy.

When creating an action plan, you want it to be easy, comfortable, and sustainable. From personal experience and helping many others to better health, it often comes down to choosing just one thing to work on, not many.

I've yet to meet someone who refuses to do anything. There's often something that person likes to do that moves them towards better bodily stewardship. For me, it's CrossFit because it demands intensity and my full effort to get results, and I do it first thing in the morning when I can give my *best* 10%. When I'm diligent and structured with that routine, other aspects of health and leadership development fall into place better. I read my Bible more consistently. I journal more consistently. I eat better. I assess and communicate more effectively. The list goes on. When I miss a workout, my day is thrown off from the very beginning.

Always add first what you love

Behavior modification works when you *add* something you love; it doesn't work when it takes away something you love or adds something you hate.

If you *hate* exercising, *hate* 6 am, or both, then resolving to exercise is a nonstarter. But if you love hiking because it quiets your thoughts and connects you with God, then that's what you should add or add more of to your daily health routine.

You may resolve to give up bread, but you love the smell, the feeling of tearing a piece from a loaf, and you love that it reminds you of great family meals growing up. Fat chance at changing that behavior until you add something good before it. Instead of giving up bread, add a good habit—such as drinking 8 oz. of water or eating a fresh vegetable—before you eat the bread. You don't have to give up beer and pizza. Just have a salad and glass of water first as your love song to your DNA.

When you do the one thing you love that helps improve your health, it makes every other action easier. For me, it's exercise. For you it may be reading, drinking water, writing in a gratitude journal, having a consistent bedtime, shutting off your cell phone for an hour or more each day, eating dinner with your family, or something else. This may take some time to figure out. Once you do, make sure the activity you love gets your *first* and *best* 10%.

Go cold turkey on addictions

Addictions are the exceptions to adding what you love. Whether it's substance abuse, porn, over spending, or another destructive behavior, you need to cut it off ASAP and get some professional help and accountability.

Addictions are massive contradictions in your philosophy, purpose, and psychology; and they *will* cause massive destruction—usually before you are ready to face the consequences.

God has a funny way of getting our attention like that. Which brings us to perhaps the favorite addiction of too many servant leaders.

The 4-letter word you're addicted to

There's one four-letter word I hear more than any other and makes me shiver and shudder. You, too, hear this word everywhere: on network TV, from co-workers, friends, and even strangers. Maybe you use this word, and maybe you're kids are using it but you're not noticing.

But you should notice because that four-letter word is one of the most offensive and detrimental to leading your flock and to being a good steward of your body. The word is *busy*, and I even got a little angry as I typed it.

"Busy" is our society's new currency of perceived success. No longer do people brag about how much money they make or how big their house is. When someone gives me the excuse that they are too busy for x, y, z, I say they're right, and I ask if they know what busy means. Do you know? Here's what we find at www.merriam-webstser.com:

BUSY: ...FOOLISHLY OR INTRUSIVELY ACTIVE...

In his book, *Addicted to Busy,* Brady Boyd says "Ultimately, every problem I see in every person I know is a problem of moving too fast for too long in too many aspects of life."

People may complain about the rush of life but they rarely do anything about it.

Why do busy (foolishly active) people have a hard time with healthy discipline? Because being busy releases dopamine, a pleasure and reward hormone. The need for speed—or more accurately, dopamine—is addicting.

Like all humans, you have a neurological need for speed. Your nervous system has the prime role of organizing and coordinating your life experiences between two categories: survival and protection, or growth and repair. I'll be referring to those two modes a lot in this book, so from here forward, I'll use the short terms "protection" and "growth," with some occasional exceptions.

Now, drill this into your head: You are always in one mode or the other; you cannot be in both modes at the same time. Dr. Bruce Lipton, PhD, author of *The Biology of Belief,* opened my eyes to this fact.

You should be able to switch back and forth, easily and efficiently, between protection and growth. But when one mode gets used more than the other, the more frequently used one becomes our default setting. The busy person often has a default setting of protection. Physiologically, this is the fight-or-flight side—what I sometimes call the "gas pedal"—of life. What do you use the gas pedal for? To go fast. Going fast isn't the problem. Like Boyd said, the problem is going too fast for too long in too many directions. If you have the gas pedal floored in your car for too long, there are two potential outcomes: crash and crash hard or burn out and run out of gas.

Busyness is not a victimless crime. Your busyness will destroy your effectiveness as a leader while hurting the people who should matter most. To get going again, your only solution is to build up your brake pedal so you're better equipped to slow down, refuel, and make sure everyone around you is safe.

To build up your brake pedal, you need to pursue healthy strategies for taking care of yourself. You need to find the brake pedal before the brake pedal finds you. I referenced it earlier in Chapter 1, but it deserves a second look.

> *If we do not allow for a rhythm of rest in our overly busy lives, illness becomes our Sabbath - our pneumonia, our cancer, our heart attack, our accidents create Sabbath for us.*—Wayne Muller

How it breaks you

In my healing leadership role, too often I see—up close and personal—how busy breaks you. It starts with chronic colds and flus, and progresses to heart issues, auto-immune issues, and hormone issues. Busyness accumulates and so does the potential damage of flooring the gas pedal without adequate brakes.

Another way that busy breaks you is through distractions. Texting while driving? That's the ultimate crashing solution to a floored gas pedal.

So what do distractions look like for leaders? Distractions are the things that are overtly contradictory to one's values.

Well-known church leaders caught up in extra marital affairs and porn. Top physical athletes with drug and alcohol addictions. People who appear to have it all and commit suicide.

And servant leaders who have broken spirits. Like hostages, they are kept in a constant state of mental and physical fatigue by being denied rest, and eventually they lose the "why" of their missions. In this case, servant leaders do it to themselves: they are captors torturing themselves and their missions by torturing their health.

How to break it

Breaking busy is a condition of your personal freedom. Be free. Start by being your true self, ditching your smart phone, and eating with your family. Enjoy your own quiet time and give your brain space to heal.

Be your true self. The more I went to seminars and conferences on success, the more I wanted to be like the guys on stage. I kept failing at trying to be those people so I stopped going to those types of events. Honestly, relative to breaking busy, it was *the* best decision I made because it compelled me to recognize my own success. I was forced to get to know and be *me*.

A problem for many of us is that we use busyness to distract ourselves from ourselves. We're not sure we like who we are. We're not sure we're good enough. We spend precious time comparing ourselves to others.

As leaders, we exhaust ourselves by always striving to do more and do better. It's easier to find rest when the only person you are comparing yourself to is yourself.

Teddy Roosevelt gets credit for saying, "Comparison is the thief of joy." I give credit to Rory Vaden, author of *Take the Stairs*, for driving that point into my head, and to Sally Hogshead for driving it into my *soul*.

In her book, *How the World Sees You*, she says, "The greatest value you can add is to become more of you," and your greatest value is what others find fascinating about you. Sally's is a very different approach than other personal assessment methods. Here's a summary of what I discovered about myself.

The world sees me as:

having a quiet demeanor and strong inner core;

being independent and self-reliant;

taking a rational approach to problem solving;

basing decisions on hard data and not gut feeling;

confident of finding solutions and reaching goals.

My *best* ways to add value (behaviors that the world will appreciate and will fuel me) are to:

set high goals;

use methodologies to reach my goals;

approach objectives in a focused, systematic way;

avoid forceful pushing or overt shows of strength;

lead in a understated way;

show others how a job is done;

mentor by explaining processes step-by-step.

My *least* effective ways to add value (behaviors that the world will not appreciate and will drain me) is to:

try to be the life of the party;

try to be a natural networker;

rush in getting to know others.

Of all the personality assessments out there from Meyers-Briggs to DISC, *How the World Sees Me* is by far the one that helped me understand *me* the best. In fact, it's freaky how accurate the descriptions are. I remember reading it to my team while they sat there nodding their heads and smiling in agreement. Once I understood what parts of me will fascinate, I stopped trying to mimic the parts of the "big guys" that drained me.

To find out more, read or listen to her book, *How the World Sees You: Discover Your Highest Value Through the Science of Fascination.* The book or audio should have a code listed with it that you can use to take the assessment for free. Or, you don't have a code, you can also buy the assessment at http://www.howtofascinate.com/.

Ditch the smart phones. People are so attached to FOMO (fear of missing out). Here's the irony: go to any playground and I guarantee that 70% of the parents have their eyes glued to their phone screens. So what they are actually missing out on is their kid.

It's amazing how much time is saved when not looking at a screen. It's amazing how you can connect with people when you don't feel the need to pull the computer out of your pocket anytime you have to wait longer than 30 seconds. If you value "real life" more than the phone alert, then put the phone away; let *it* wait for you.

The next time you're in the airport, put the phone down and just watch all the other people on their phones. People say that zombies are coming. I say they are already here.

Eat dinner together. Just search online for "stats of eating meals together" and have fun reading. We never made dinner a ritual for the reasons reported in the statistics, but it's nice to know our dinners are not only feeding our kids nutritionally but also relationally, emotionally, and sometimes comically.

When I say dinner together, it's actually at a dining room table, TV off, and no phones. We do put music on but it's not a distraction to us unless one of the kids gets jiggy with it and spills something.

Add a deadline-free quiet activity. Reading or listening to music by yourself are classic examples of adding quiet activity to your life. If you don't want to do more Bible reading and are too busy to research something else to read, then I have a suggestion: Steven Covey's *The 7 Habits of Highly Effective People*, and focus on the urgent vs. important concepts. Notice it's not titled the 453 tasks of overly busy people?

As weird as it may sound, cleaning a pool is one of the most relaxing things I do. I love being around the calm water, moving slowly, and not having a deadline—especially now that I know the origins of the word:

The term deadline originally referred to a physical

line in a prison camp. Prisoners who stepped over
the line were shot.—http://www.etymonline.com/

Find a quiet activity that breaks your busy. Make it something that serves others while serving you. In my case, cleaning the pool earns brownie points with the in-laws.

You now know four easy things you can do to start breaking busy. Notice the list does not include sleeping more or
vegging out. It does include behaviors that can recharge
you—and that won't kill you in the process.

Your procedures action plan

Your habits are your procedures. Whether you choose to continue living with poor habits vs. mastering good habits won't
affect your salvation, but it will affect your leadership effectiveness and definitely call into question whether you are, in
fact, being a good steward of God's gift: your body.

Let's assume you choose to be a good steward. Here are
your next steps.

1. List the three things you won't give up. This is your safe
   zone in sustainable, stewardship change.

2. List three things you *love* to do that you consider healthy.
   Then choose one to add to your day and schedule it when
   you can give your best and first 10% of effort.

3. Once the one thing you love to do is habit, repeat step
   two, and add another thing.

Commit to breaking busy in small steps:

• Make a *To Be* list based on your *true* self.

- Work on your *To Be* list before your *To Do* list.

- Replace your smart phone with a less intrusive one.

- Schedule one TV-free meal a day with family.

- Do deadline-free, quiet activities.

CHAPTER 5

GET MORE DONE BY SETTING BOUNDARIES ON DOING

I think the single biggest impact on my leadership development happened early in my career. I was a year out of school with great ambitions of saving this planet from needless suffering and ailments from chronic conditions.

No matter how much I worked, how many people I helped, I felt inadequate. Instead of comparing me to me, I was comparing my efforts and results to others who I perceived as more successful.

At the time my girlfriend (now my wife) was working at Compassion International. She was an assistant to the executive VP and went on many leadership retreats with the executive team, including attending the Willow Creek Leadership Summit every year.

In 2006, after returning from a Summit event, she gave me an audio recording of "a guy you're going to love." She was right. The speaker on the recording forever changed my life and set me up to break busy before busy broke me.

Though you may not have known me before reading this book, you probably do know of the man who did so much to shape how I approach leadership and health stewardship: Andy Stanley, leader of North Point Community Church in Georgia, son of Charles Stanley, author, and many other roles...but I'm not comparing.

During that Leadership Summit, he spoke of his "greatest leadership decision ever." Andy Stanley did something that I thought was impossible: he made a deal with God. Andy explained it like this:

> *God, I don't have time to build a ministry and take care of my family. I'll give you 45 hours per week as a church planter. If you can build a church on 45 hours, I'm your guy. I'll let you build as big a church as you can with that 45 hours, and I'll be satisfied with that. But I'm not going to cheat my family.*

The deal worked. Today, Andy's North Point Ministries serve over 15,000 people every Sunday. He even closes his church the last Sunday of December to give the staff time off. There was some controversy over this a few years back when that last Sunday landed on Christmas day.

No church on Christmas? He almost got hung for heresy in some Christian circles. But he was congruent with his values; that's successful leadership. He had his 4 Ps aligned.

Andy's message of having faith in God to expand the ministry—or any other specific venture—and not feeling guilty about taking time for Andy was so freeing for me, especially as a young professional.

GET MORE DONE BY SETTING BOUNDARIES ON DOING **61**

It was the first time I heard it's okay to put boundaries on your mission. It's okay to *not* put in 70 hours per week for fear of not reaching that next person. It's okay to have a great mission *and* have a great home life; and, in fact, only by having both can you have a life where your philosophy, purpose, psychology, and procedures are congruent. There was no need to continue running myself into the ground with the war cry "It's for a good cause!"

Andy Stanley went on to say that our calling isn't necessarily our mission, citing Ephesians 5:25:

> *Husbands, love your wives, just as Christ loved the church and gave himself up for her.*

If there was a downside to hearing Andy's message it was my hard realization that the servant leaders in my life were hostages to their missions. They were completely giving themselves up for their mission, instead of keeping some reserves to love their spouse, kids, and family.

We get sucked into thinking that we are called to build our church, business, or career, and with prayer that God alone will take care of our family. It's actually the opposite way. We are called to love and take care of our family and allow God to build the mission.

There will be seasons of increased work load and mission focused duties but at the end of life are you going to wish you spent more time leading or more time enjoying and taking care of your family? Make sure you recognize that season and make sure it is temporary.

After hearing Andy's message, I immediately read his

book, *Visioneering*, another must read for the leader; there's a chapter in the book on distractions. Recall that in Chapter 4 in this book, I described how distractions are a key way that busy breaks you. I painted a negative picture of addictions like affairs, distractions, and even suicide.

Sometimes those distractions are masked in an entirely different wrapping: a shiny package of opportunity. This has potential to increase your busy factor by 100 fold and you don't realize what is happening.

Inevitably, these opportunities arrive just when you're feeling successful at breaking busy and truly caring for your family. You're finally connecting by spending uninterrupted time together; by having dinner together, getting crazy with each other with laughs, giggles, and wrestling in the 60-90 minutes between dinner and bedtime, and then tucking in with prayer.

I'm not saying you have to be home every night for dinner and bedtime. With industries working around the clock, you may have to make a different pattern of family time. Maybe it's making sure you have breakfast each morning before the kids go to school and you head off to the office. I foresee this happening in my own home—trading evening connections for morning connections—as my kids get older and involved with sports and other activities that are more evening centric.

Just set a limit, like Andy Stanley, to be used by God. There are 168 hours in a week; if you give God 45, then you'll still have 123 hours each week to take care of you and your family. (Sleep counts as taking care of you!)

Assess if you're a hostage to your mission. Being called to

take care of your family, means taking care of yourself so you have enough fuel in your tank to serve and provide for them.

It's like the airplane oxygen mask. Put your mask on first before trying to help someone else. If you're in a coma, you're no good to anyone else.

By the way, my retelling of Andy Stanley's message does not do it justice. I urge you to dig up a CD or DVD recording of the 2006 Willow Creek Leadership Summit and keep listening to it until you've worn it to the point it skips. I admit it can be hard to find, so if your library doesn't carry it ask about an interlibrary loan. Amazon or eBay are other possible sources. Search on these phrases: "The Leadership Summit 2006 Team Edition" and "Focused Leadership Andy Stanley."

PART II

DEVELOPING A CULTURE OF PERSONAL HEALTH

If you're a church leader reading this, then I ask: What's the number one prayer request? Many of your peers would say prayers to help their congregations cope with health issues.

If you're a business leader, what is the fastest growing expense in your organization? Employee health insurance... assuming you're still offering it instead of abandoning it as many other companies have.

If you're a financial planner, attorney, or irs employee, what's the number one cause of personal bankruptcy that you see? Medical costs.

I have a bold suggestion: By developing a culture of personal health we will have more time and money available to spend on fulfilling personal, family, and organizational missions. The resources we spend in creating health will be resources spent well.

Developing a culture of personal health does take patience and courage. Just as there are no legitimate "get rich, quick" programs, there are no "get healthy, quick" programs. However, there's plenty you can do to start momentum. It's a big topic, so we'll cover it in several chapters. We'll start with the idea of being a health leader; then we'll move to body science; and the food vices you need to confront. Then you'll be ready for Part III, your 7 Day Jump Start to Health.

CHAPTER 6

BEING A STEWARD LEADER OF HEALTH

You may have heard the quote from leadership expert, Pastor John Maxwell, "Leadership is Influence, nothing more, nothing less." In other words, leaders have influence and leaders are influencers.

According to the top search results in Google, influence is the capacity to have an effect on the character, development, or behavior of someone or something.

There's physical influence like when you steer a car. You have the influence to keep that vehicle straight down the highway or you have the influence to spontaneously jerk the wheel into head on traffic.

There's chemical influence like what you feed your kids. You can affect their development or behavior by choosing to feed them vegetables versus feeding them Pixie Sticks.

And there's financial influence. We've all seen the influence money brings when groups lobby on Capitol Hill. According to the Center for Responsive Politics (www.opensecrets.org), between 1998-2015 the pharmaceutical/health products industry spent $3.25 billion on lobbyists, with $2.1 billion (almost 65%) from the pharmaceutical manufacturing sector. That's *a lot* of spending to influence our nation's decision makers.

If leadership is influence, does being influential make you a leader? In parenting, a baby influences parental behavior, but is hardly a leader. A baby cries or poops, mom and dad jump to the rescue. A baby falls asleep on your chest; you don't move an inch.

Leading others by leading yourself

"Steward leadership" connotes two ideas:

- That your leadership influence should have a positive effect on the character, development, or behavior of someone.

- The person most influenced should be you. By being a steward, you are leading yourself to a better version of you, physically, chemically, emotionally, spiritually, and socially.

Let's take a closer look at each idea.

You're a leader until they decide you're not

"Which way did they go? I must find them. I am their leader!"—Alexandre Ledru-Rollin, French politician, 1848

How do we judge leadership in today's culture? A person's influence can certainly be measured by how many people are impacted by their mission, business, TV or radio show, or by how much money they give away or amass. These are all great snapshot measurements, but here's the bitter truth: leadership and influence can be taken away from the leader in an instant.

This goes back to breaking busy. If you don't break busy, then it breaks you with its crashes or distractions. Not surprisingly, it's their crashes and distractions that often cause us to "unfollow" the people we used to admire and aspire to be like.

Whatever the scenario—the athlete taking PEDS (performance enhancing drugs), the senator caught in an extramarital affair, or something else—leaders are judged harshest by our actions, not by our words. More is caught than taught.

If you want to be a great steward leader, you have to realize you're a role model first for your family, and then for the rest of your flock. Your family is first because you have the most influence over them; they see you at your highest highs and lowest lows; they're the ones who will (or won't) attend your funeral; and when they lead others, they'll either choose to lead in a way that resembles how you led, or they'll say "I'm never doing it like that."

Christian author, Max Lucado, tweeted, "Ponder your success and count your money in a cemetery, and remember that neither of the two is buried with you."

Max Lucado @MaxLucado · 3h
Ponder your success and count your money in a cemetery, and remember-
neither of the two is buried with you.

    160   210   · · ·

In other words, on your deathbed, you're never going to look back and regret serving more people. You will, however, regret not serving your family better. The best way to serve them is by making sure you're serving yourself first.

If you can't influence yourself, how do you expect to influence those around you? When parents insist, "I can't get my kids to eat vegetables," I respond, "It's hard; I can't get my toddler son, Lukas, to stop smoking at the dinner table."

After a funny look, they ask, "What do you mean?"

"Are you eating your vegetables?" I ask.

Mom or dad usually doesn't say much after that. You can't expect someone else to *do* something that you aren't willing to do yourself. You can't expect people to *be* something unless you're willing to be it yourself. In addition to setting a good example, we have to eliminate the "bad" options for them to choose. Rather than "What do you want for breakfast," ask the kids, "Would you prefer eggs or oatmeal for breakfast today?" For most kids, hunger will set in eventually and they will eat the good choices you have available... they won't die by failing to eat mac and cheese today.

If you don't take time to connect with your kids when they are young, don't expect your kids to take time to connect with you when you're old.

Influencing yourself is tricky business

A few paragraphs earlier, I noted that, more than anyone, steward leaders should have a positive influence on themselves. Here's the tricky part: we influence ourselves by the way we respond to expectations, and by our courage.

Expectation innies and outies

In her book, *Better Than Before: Mastering the Habits of Our Everyday Lives*, Gretchen Rubin notes that people respond differently to inner and outer expectations. Outer expectations are what's expected of us, such as meeting work deadlines; inner expectations are what we expect or desire for ourselves, such as being a healthy steward leader.

Rubin breaks down how people respond into four categories: Upholders (a small minority); Questioners, and Obligers (most common); and Rebels (a larger minority).

Upholders are people who respond well to inner AND outer expectations without much effort.

Questioners question all expectations. They do something if it makes sense. If your expectation seems arbitrary or irrational, they want to know *why* they should listen to you. Questioners make everything an inner expectation.

Obligers readily meet outward expectations but struggle mightily to meet inner expectations. If they are on a team or have a coach, they easily complete the task at hand. Obligers hire coaches when they want to run marathons. They follow the training plan exactly, eating, running, and resting as prescribed. But after the race is over and there's no more coaching or plan to follow, they never run again.

Rebels, on the other hand, want to do it their way on their schedule, and the way they see best. The more you tell them to do something, the more they will do the opposite. Even though people who are overarching Rebels are a minority, I think we all have a little rebel in us, especially in a marriage. For example, our spouse wants something done a certain way. We rebel and do it our way. The task gets done but conflict arises because our process wasn't their process.

I've discovered that I'm a Questioner. If I know the sensible *why* behind something, then I'm usually good to go. I think this is why the 4 Ps matter so much to me. When I understand the philosophy, purpose, and psychology behind my procedures (what I do) then I can make realistic, intentional, and to-the-point changes to lead myself in a manner that allows me to lead others for a long and effective time. Being a questioner is also probably why I subscribe to "beliefs dictate behaviors."

For a snapshot of how you respond to inner and outer expectations, take the quiz at www.GretchenRubin.com.

Courage and fear are in the job requirements

Regardless of who you are leading—a mega church, your family, or just yourself—and you're being successful, then there's fear and courage involved. Fear creates *inaction*. Courage doesn't mean you aren't scared to lead and be a good steward. Courage just means you are doing more than making decisions; you are *taking actions* for your organization.

Dale Partridge, the CEO of Sevenly and the Wall Street Journal best-selling author of *People Over Profits*, says of leadership, "It's your job to remember. It's your job to be disciplined. It's your job to be consistent and to stand up."

This is why I'm so passionate about leaders taking care of themselves. If you, as a leader, don't create discipline, maturity, and the ability to stand strong when it comes to your own health, then your leadership effectiveness goes out the window, and your family will suffer the most.

So I admit I'm sensitive to this topic, having seen the men in my family lead so hard for others that they didn't have enough in their tanks, long term, for themselves or their families.

The easiest way for you to put enough in your tank to be a steward leader is to muster the courage be healthy.

Having the courage to be healthy

One of the traits separating leaders from others is courage. Courage doesn't mean you aren't afraid, nervous, or worried. It means you are taking action despite being afraid, nervous, or worried. Courage can also mean *not* conforming.

Whether you are a religious, business, government, or home leader, ask yourself: do my followers have health courage? If they don't have courage, what can I do to help them get it?

Here's a suggestion: Stop celebrating what's wrong. Start celebrating what's right, and start being an example of how to build health.

Stop celebrating disease, drugs, and destructive messages

How are ailments celebrated? With drugs and destructive messages. "Managing" chronic illness is one of the destructive messages deeply ingrained in our healthcare system. Another destructive message is to look for an event as the cause of a problem. If your doctors can't find a direct event, then the illness gets chalked up to genetics, family history, old age, or being part of the unlucky club.

Perhaps the most pervasive and destructive messages of all are the commercials and advertisements that show people who—despite their chronic illnesses—are really happy, thanks to the doling out of drugs and more drugs.

DON'T BE ASHAMED; CELEBRATE YOUR ADHD, YOUR DIABETES, YOUR LUPUS, YOUR MENTAL HEALTH DISEASE, AND ALL OF YOUR OTHER AILMENTS! AND LISTEN TO THE HAPPY MUSIC WE'VE ADDED SO YOU WON'T PAY TOO MUCH ATTENTION TO THE WARNINGS; BECAUSE IF YOU REALLY PAID ATTENTION, YOU MIGHT QUESTION WHY THE DRUG COULD MAKE YOUR CONDITION WORSE OR KILL YOU.

What if we changed the scenario and started celebrating debt? What if we celebrated divorce? What if we celebrated drug addiction? What if we celebrated violence?

Oh, wait. We already do with media coverage. And what's the result? More debt, more divorce, more drug addiction, and more violence.

Ironically, even those "walks for awareness" of ABC disease indirectly celebrate illness because even as early detection and treatment for conditions like depression, arthritis, and Alzheimer's skyrocket, so do the disabilities associated with those ailments.

Here's an example. In his book, *Anatomy of an Epidemic*, Robert Whitaker states:

The rise in the number of disabled mentally ill has been especially pronounced since 1987, the year that Prozac, the first of the "second-generation" psychiatric drugs, arrived on the market. The number of adults on SSI or SSDI due to mental illness has risen from 1.25 million in 1987 to more than 4 million today. The number of children and youth on SSI due to a serious mental illness has skyrocketed from 16,200 in 1987 to more than 600,000 today.

If we keep celebrating people's ailments with drugs and destructive messages, there's no way people will get healthier. It's time to *stop* celebrating disease. When we celebrate disease instead of tackling it by building health, we enable people to stay comfortable while they die quicker. If your congregation or organizational members stay sick, you soon won't have anyone to lead.

Start celebrating health courage

Was FDR elected four times because he celebrated his paralysis? No. He was elected for showing leadership and strength.

As a leader you can show health leadership and strength. Stop celebrating disease and drugs and start developing a personal culture of health by doing three things:

- Stop lying to yourself that your suffering will bring healing to others.

- Start adding health to your daily routine. For simple, small steps you can start tomorrow, see the *7-Day Jump*

Start to Health that I've included in this book.

- When you have a setback on your way to health, celebrate failure. Yes, you read that right.

Developing a culture of personal health is scary for a lot of people, and it may be scary for you. The fear stems in part from the sheer quantity of information and choices available.

It seems odd that anyone would fear doing something that has no downside, but it can happen with health the same as it does for debt. Large debt can paralyze people with inaction; so they stay in debt their whole lives or go even further into debt.

But it's better to try fifty times and fail than to never try. As Ryan Holiday, the young entrepreneur and author of *The Obstacle is the Way*, says, "Failure shows us the way by showing us what isn't the way."

So if you have setbacks on your way to health, I want you to *celebrate*. Be proud; you took action and because now you know what *not* to do; you've narrowed your health options and improved your focus. So, if you take away anything from this book, let it be this:

- Courage is action.

- Faith without action is dead.

- Action is easier when your 4 Ps are aligned because what you do is tied to a mission larger than yourself.

There's something in particular you'll need to have a lot of courage to do for yourself: break the vices that put your health in a vice.

Leader vices that put health in a vice

For leaders, I see some common cultural health practices that *will* affect your ability to lead: busyness and building community with food.

We covered the perils of busyness and how to break it before it breaks you in Part I. Here we'll introduce the food aspect and then cover it in detail in the next chapter

Building community with food

I grew up in an ultra conservative church: no dancing, no guitars, and definitely no food in the sanctuary. We had to have some way of building community, and potlucks were it.

When I left home and found my new church family in different parts of the country, I found a different community-building culture. Along with potlucks, every church had it's own café offering specialty coffee beverages and a generous spread of pastries and cakes.

No matter how conservative or charismatic the church, there's one thing that brings church folk into community almost more than loving Jesus...loving food.

Three foods that ill and kill community

Whether it's potluck or the church café, three staples seem to be in endless supply: caffeine, wheat, and sugar. These three church staples are also likely the biggest contributors to the prayer requests you receive on a weekly basis, and the biggest threat to your longevity as a leader.

The thought of not having caffeine, wheat, and sugar to build community might be more stressful than getting the bill to replace smoking brakes. But here's what I can assure you: regular consumption of caffeine, wheat, and sugar will seriously smoke your body brakes, your wallet, and eventually your leadership effectiveness. Here's why: When routinely ingested, caffeine, wheat, and sugar will shift your physiology to default protection mode. The longer you're there, the more likely you'll have an exponential increase in toxicities and deficiencies that lead to the greatest brakesmoking situation of all: chronic illness and disease outcomes.

In the next chapters, I'll explain more about the effects of your food choices. But first, let's get back to philosophy, the first of the 4 Ps because your food choices are, after all, guided by your metaphysical view of where health comes from.

Fair warning: you'll notice I pick on wheat a lot and say little about corn, rice, and other grains. This book is about the start of a health journey; it's not *the* journey. I chose wheat to get you started. So don't think that reducing or eliminating your wheat intake is a greenlight for chowing down on anything gluten-free. If you have health problems, then expect to be disappointed when gluten-free is not your panacea. If you're serious about understanding the effects of all grains, then read *Grain Brain* by David Perlmutter, MD (a book I mention again in a later chapter).

CHAPTER 7

WHERE DOES HEALTH COME FROM?

Health is not as complex as drug companies, politicians, and others would have us believe. Health is simple. God put certain health requirements into your DNA, and your DNA depends on you to meet those requirements. God also put certain *non*-requirements into your DNA, and your DNA depends on you to stay away from those things.

God also gave us limbs and the ability to reason so we could hunt, forage, and teach the next generation to do the same things. Scriptures tell us that He also gave us instructions to take care of things, including ourselves.

As Christians, we know that it's not one but often a series of many temptations that lead someone further and further from God until one day they wake up realizing they are addicted to porn and facing a divorce. We also know that to be forgiven and redeemed of our sins, we have to create action that leads us back to sufficiency and purity. Our health journey is no different. It's a journey that created ill health, and it's a journey to regain it.

Fatalist, DNAist, or Stewardist?

Imagine you are on the high school debate team and you must defend your answer to the question, "Where does health come from?" You must take the position of a Fatalist, DNAist, or Stewardist, and your arguments must be consistent with your Christian views. Here's how the debate plays out.

The Fatalist. If you believe God is solely responsible for your health then you are asserting beliefs such as these:

- You have no free agency because if God is pleased with you, then you have health. If God is not pleased, then you get disease. Your choices to remedy the situation don't matter.

- You are not blessed to be a Christian. If God is the dictator of health, then why do people of other religions, agnostics, and atheists also experience great health?

The DNAist. If you believe your health is only in your DNA then you are asserting beliefs such as these:

- You have free agency to abuse your body because your DNA guarantees you either a healthy life or an illness-filled life. Your choices to remedy illness won't matter because you are in the lucky or the unlucky club.

- Your DNA—not your Christian behavior—is the reason you feel better when you are grateful, forgiving, eating clean, and exercising regularly; and why you feel grumpy, bitter, or hateful after gorging on cake, cigarettes, NFL games, and (un)reality TV shows.

You may also find it difficult to explain why identical twins—people who have the *same* DNA—can have totally different health outcomes.

The Stewardist. If your answer is "from God and from me," then you'll have an easier time of defending your views because you don't have contradictions in your approach to health. You are asserting that by taking charge of your health you are asserting that:

- You have free agency; your health choices matter.

- Caring for yourself is being obedient: to be a good steward of God's creation.

Health algebra and plastic nervous systems

If you're a health Stewardist then, in addition to being a free agent, you "get" the math. Expressed as algebra, it looks like this:

$$constants \ (God + your \ {\scriptsize DNA}) + variable \ ({\scriptsize YOU}) = health$$

The variable that affects your health is *you* making health choices every day, all day. Your choices affect how your DNA interacts with your nervous system that, as you'll recall, flip-flops within microseconds between protection and growth mode; you can never be in both modes at once.

Finding a balance so you're not stuck in one mode or the other is essential. If you're chronically ill, your nervous system is most likely stuck in survival and protection because that's what your body will always favor. Though you'll seldom hear about it, getting stuck in growth and repair can happen, too, and that's a problem because it means your body is not being sufficiently challenged; like a newborn baby you have no defenses. You need to be in protection at times so you can build your defenses.

I do see people who are stuck in repair mode. Sadly, it's people who have pretty much used all their survival capabilities and are burned out. I also see people stuck in repair mode due to medication. Many drugs like antidepressants, antipsychotics, and muscle relaxers are suppressing the nervous system's ability to go into survival mode.

To put it in context, if you're stuck in repair mode, whether due to burn out or medication-induced suppression of your survival side, then you have no way of escaping the bear. You may see the bear and try to give it a hug.

Luckily, God gave you a plastic nervous system so you can regain your health; you don't have to stay stuck. Like bending the flat handle of a plastic spoon into a curved handle, you can bend your mind and body so you can become a better steward of your health. When you bend the spoon too fast, you are giving it too much input too fast, and it breaks. But bend it slowly with consistency and repetition, and you can mold that flat handle into a curved one and make the curved handle the default.

Our nervous systems are no different. The area with the most consistent and repeated input becomes our default pathway for either growth or protection mode. In the next part, I'll use two examples—bears and wilted plants—to further explain how our nervous systems work and how they respond to the wrong versus right kind of care.

When bears attack...

Imagine we're taking a 14 mile hike up Pikes Peak. Stopping for a break to enjoy the beauty God created, a light breeze whips up, cooling our faces.

You spot a small stream and walk towards it to listen more closely to its peaceful running water. The breeze picks up, flying leaves by your head. We both start laughing, and behind-the-scene our nervous systems are in growth mode.

Then, in a spare second, you see a bear blocking you from heading back to the trail. Instantly, your nervous system switches to protection mode, preparing to defend itself.

Your heart is racing, blood pressure pounding, and muscles firing in case you need to flee or fight your way out. And then, lucky you! A fish jumps in the stream, distracting the bear, and leaving you to walk slowly back to the trail.

The coast clear, we continue our hike. We come to another great spot, drop our daypacks, and grab a snack. A half hour later, you've calmed down and momentarily forgotten your bear encounter. Ever the stream-lover, you spot another and leave the trail to check it out. Your nervous system has switched back to growth mode.

Again, the wind picks up, circling leaves around your head, and smacking a few against your ears. "Not again," you say with lighthearted exasperation. You turn from the stream and there's another bear between you and the trail. You're back in protection mode.

Just like the first time, a fish jumps in the stream, distracting the bear from you and to some bear fishing, giving you a chance to back away. Compared to the first time, you're walking slower even though your heart is pounding harder. You're also feeling light headed and queasy because you've escaped two potentially dangerous situations within a fairly short time.

You say you're fine and we continue our hike. By now you've decided that the next time you see a stream, no matter how enticing, you're not going near it.

We stay on the trail, but the wind didn't get the memo. It picks up, swirling leaves around your head. You jerk around to make sure no bear behind you. You're safe. But then a squirrel darts across your boot, putting you into full survival and protection (a.k.a. panic) mode.

You return home and visit your doctor for a checkup. You're told your blood pressure is elevated, cholesterol is up, and testosterone is down. Though all-out panic has passed, your nervous system is still *stressed* and in protection mode. Your doctor prescribes drugs, and so you enter the cycle of "healthcare" that seeks to cover symptoms, rather than finding and curing the underlying causes. Your doctor didn't know your bear story, and if they did, they might still have prescribed drugs.

The bear story illustrates how our bodies switch between growth and protection mode; how we get stuck in protection; and how the healthcare system keeps us there.

For leaders from top level executives to the stay-at-home moms, *stress* is the bear that propels our bodies into protection mode. With repeated stressors—whether physical, chemical, emotional, spiritual, or social—and no time off to heal and repair, our systems default into protection mode. In the next topic, I explain more about how our nervous systems work, and what happens when it's always in protection mode.

Our bodies react...

God created our nervous systems to coordinate and organize our life experiences into protection or growth "memories." When something happens to trigger a memory, your nervous system sends messengers (hormones) to your DNA. Your DNA responds by producing a protein code so that your body responds appropriately.

Let's say that bear did attack you and you're bleeding. From nervous system to DNA to protein code to action, your body physiologically responds by increasing your clotting factors to keep you from bleeding to death. Short term, clotting is a great thing. Long term, clots kill you.

Similarly, in sustained protection mode, your body experiences chronic levels of stressors—deficiencies and toxicities—which lead to a host of physiological responses that shift and stay that way. So over time, a pounding heart, sweaty palms, poor digestion, and more protection responses become your body's default. And that leads to plundered health in the form of chronic illness and disease.

Inflammation is normal; sustained inflammation isn't

God created the body intelligently. The body never does stupid things; we do. Any reaction in the body in response to a stress is the body's intelligent adaptation to buy you enough time to escape the stress.

It's our stupidity for not recognizing this and "treating" intelligent, adaptive stress by adding more stress. There's only so much time before the body gets fatigued and chronic stress sets in.

Adaptive INTELLIGENT responses to stress	Consequences of CHRONIC stress
blood pressure increases	heart attack
heart rate increases	heart disease
cholesterol increases (LDL up, HDL down)	stroke
respiration gets faster	chronic obstructive pulmonary disease (COPD)
clotting factors increase	stroke • embolism
blood sugars increase	diabetes • obesity • behavior changes such as being over-active
insulin resistance increases	diabetes • cancers • polycystic ovary syndrome (PCOS) • hormone imbalances • Alzheimer's
sensitivity to your surroundings increases	ADHD • autism • dementia

(learning, memory, and concentration decrease) |
immune system has an imbalance (antibodies are dominant)	autoimmune conditions like MS, rheumatoid arthritis, lupus, IBS, Crohn's disease, Type 1 diabetes
muscle tension and contraction increases	chronic fatigue • fibromyalgia • chronic pain
digestion decreases	GERD • acid reflux • IBS
fertility decreases	hormone imbalances • miscarriages
thyroid decreases	changes in metabolism, mood, and fetal development

And that was the short list.

If you've been diagnosed with a chronic condition, then you're using Visa to pay off AmEx, and AmEx to pay off Discover, and Discover to pay off Diner's Card from 1983. In other words, chronic illness is the result of your body adapting itself to death.

No bear repellent here: Drugs, surgery, and enablers

Our healthcare system is not set up to achieve health by preventing or curing chronic conditions; instead, it equates health based on detecting and managing symptoms. Fewer symptoms equate to better health. So doctors dispense—and insurance companies pay for—drugs to help you cope with symptoms, and not to actually cure you. It's like Congress increasing the debt ceiling instead of addressing entitlement programs and wasteful spending. Drugs are a short term solution to make you feel better while the underlying problems continue to build.

Symptoms—pounding heart, sweaty palms—are your body's *intelligent adaptation* to survival and protection. Imagine being on a blood pressure drug, a blood thinner, and mood stabilizer when that bear is attacking you. You may feel better on those meds but now your body can't react to get away from the bear because the drugs are suppressing your intelligent adaptation to stress. Those meds made your "numbers look good" at the expense of your long-term survival. You couldn't care less if the bear is gnawing on your leg because, on meds, you don't feel a thing.

Whatever your leadership role—pastor, parent, philanthropist, or something else—you need to get to the root problems of your health, just as you do the root problems that hinder accomplishing your mission. You know that when you identify a problem but only cover the symptoms that the problem still exists. This is called enabling.

If an alcoholic is having a hangover, you don't give him another drink to make him feel better. But this is exactly how our healthcare system works. You've seen the commercials:

"Before you belly up to those cheesy, gravy fries, corn dog, and beer that your body is violently rejecting in the form of heart burn, take these purple pills so you can destroy your body more comfortably."

The healthcare system is a system of disabling enablers.

When drugs and surgery make sense

There *is* a time and a place for drugs and surgery. Those are emergency interventions. If the bear gets you or me, you better believe I'm in favor of the pain meds and surgery to patch us back together.

Lessons from wilting plants

Where should you start on your health journey? Let's start with the concept of a wilting plant. Your leadership responsibility is to nurse this plant from its chronic illness back to a thriving state.

You innately know that the plant can get better with *appropriate* care. It would be inappropriate—and ridiculous—to paint the leaves green and use sticks to prop up the bent stalks; doing so would only mask the true dysfunction, no matter how good it looks.

You know the wilting plant has certain requirements to get and stay healthy. It needs some combination of water, sunlight, and nutrients. You also know that healing is a *process* for your plant, not an event. So you give it appropriate care, and over time you see the leaves returning to their natural color and getting bigger, and the stalks supporting the weight of the plant.

Now that you have a healthy plant, you want to maintain its health. What do you give it? The same things you used to heal it: water, sunlight, and nutrients.

This is where science and marketing create a bad health-care system because the focus is on maintaining an individual's health status quo versus *regaining* health. Yet, if you're chronically ill, you have the same requirements to get back to health as if you're already healthy and want to maintain it. You just might need more of what an already healthy person has.

What if you saw the wilting plant and you put little diesel fuel pills in the soil, a chlorophyll-lowering drug into the water, or both? What if you presented your treatment to the largest nature conservation conference in the world?

You'd be laughed off stage and Twitter trolls would blow up your profile with #PlantKiller, #GreenMeansGreen, and #BugsNotDrugs.

But if you assessed a wilting human and gave him drugs to lower cholesterol, chemotherapy to kill cells, and an inhaler to open his lungs, you're a freaking genius who gets tweets like these: #LifeSaver, #NobelPrize, and #BiPartisanPolicyChangeWeCanBelieveIn

Maybe the inmates really are running the asylum. If you're going to develop a culture of personal health, don't be an inmate.

CHAPTER 8

NERVOUS SYSTEM 101—IT'S AUTONOMIC

Your nervous system has a magic role. It has the distinct duty of organizing and coordinating what life throws at you. In split-second decisions, it organizes and coordinates your life experiences in one experience that will enhance your immediate survival and protection *or* growth and repair.

Further, your nervous system will *always* err on the side of caution and promote your internal physiology to immediate survival: survival over sex, life over legacy.

Body, mind, and drug chemistry

When you "break bread" by frantically grabbing an iced coffee grande and a danish, it can trigger the same physiological pathways as the memory of being beaten by dad as a kid. In other words, how we move and eat can create the purity and sufficiency associated with health, or the deficiencies and toxicities associated with stress.

The more stress happens, the more chronic changes in the brain happen. Stress is more than emotional strife; it can be physical, chemical, emotional, social, or spiritual strife.

Have a contradiction within your 4 Ps? That's a massive contributor to stress.

Whatever the stress, cells in the hippocampus (your learning center) literally start to shrink. Production of serotonin (a happy hormone) drops. When you add concentration and learning deficiencies on top of depression, that's a recipe for early burnout and, in my dad's case, Alzheimer's.

I first noticed it while visiting my parents a year before Dad retired. Looking for a water glass, I found his meds. Why would a pastor be on antidepressants? With that much mission and purpose in life, how can one lack joy? Sadly, Dad is a prime example of how the body can affect the mind and vice-versa, and how drugs can only make things worse.

Here's my suggestion. If you want to improve your leadership and problem solving outcomes when dealing with depression and chronic emotional issues, then address the gut: eliminate the foods that make your nervous system go haywire.

Gut instincts

Along with the rest of your body, your gut was created to keep you thriving for 120 years. Your gut consists of your stomach and intestines, a gut lining, and a delicate internal *ecosystem of bacteria* that starts in your throat and ends between your butt cheeks.

The purpose of the gut lining is to keep things within the gut, making sure that bacteria, viruses, and proteins stay in the gut and don't leak into the blood stream.

Now about that bacteria. To have a healthy immune system, you need a balance of beneficial and non-beneficial bacteria. The more bacterial imbalances, the greater the damage to your ecosystem and the gut itself. The good bacteria feeds off the good food we eat and non-beneficial bacteria feed off sugar. Eventually there's a bacterial imbalance and the gut lining is compromised. Instead of bacteria, viruses, and proteins staying put, they leak into the blood stream, putting your body into protection mode.

Why do you think so many get sick during the "flu" season? The flu season is nothing more than a sugar, wheat, and a stress orgy from Halloween, Thanksgiving, Christmas, New Year's, Valentine's Day, St. Patty's Day, and Easter. Lord, bless me with an abundance of marshmallow Peeps so I can get to Heaven sooner!

Your church potluck is filled with breads, pastas, and cookies. The foods that kids with ADHD, autism, and other sensory processing problems *always* crave are sugar and wheat products. The point is that foods consumed through a gut tube that is not intact have the potential to escape into the blood stream; a.k.a. leaky gut. Put another way, when running from a bear, you're not worried about proper digestion or elimination, which is why you experience diarrhea, queasiness, and headaches, and worse.

For the millionth time, the body will err on the side of caution and attack the "foreign" proteins. It doesn't matter if that protein is food or bacteria; it's foreign and needs to be attacked. But instead of your gut lining taking care of the problem in a quiet manner internally, a full blown immune response in the blood ensues. Part of that immune response is building antibodies against future exposure. The other part is recruiting inflammation to quarantine and destroy the invading foreign proteins.

This sets the stage for two problems. First, as more antibodies are created, they will look for anything that resembles the food protein they just attacked. In other words, the body starts building antibodies against other organs, and attacking itself. It could be brain tissue, thyroid tissue, joint tissue, or some combination of tissues. Second, inflammation loves to party. If a little inflammation is good then a lot is fantastic. Autism, Alzheimer's, Parkinson's, cancer, heart disease, obesity, and ADHD all have an inflammatory component. And, contrary as it might seem, your body is doing what it's meant to: using inflammation as an intelligent adaptation to stress.

Inflammation is intelligent adaptation

Inflammation is a *huge* word in the health and sickness industry. Everyone is blaming it for something. As much as inflammation is a contributor to *every* disease on the planet, if you couldn't produce inflammation, you wouldn't be around long enough to experience chronic illness stemming from inflammation.

Inflammation is a sure sign that your immune system is actively at work. When your immune system is healthy, then inflammation is temporary. When your system is not healthy, inflammation is chronic. If you have a chronic illness, then you have chronic inflammation.

Your body never does stupid stuff. Your body is always in a state of intelligent adaptation. Sometimes that adaptation is to produce inflammation. Inflammation happens for two life saving, life building reasons: to fight infection and to repair injured tissue.

Fight infection. This is your body's first-line defense. The coughing, sneezing, runny nose, diarrhea, fever, and sweating isn't the fault of the bug. This is your body's response to the bug. You sneeze to expel the bug at 35 mph to a distance of 12-20 feet away (according to the Myth Busters duo, who dispelled the "100 mph to 30 feet away sneeze" mantra).

Repair injured tissue. You work out to get stronger. You are also voluntarily injuring yourself for the purpose of allowing your body to build it back up again. All that soreness you experience the day or two after a workout isn't a buildup of lactic acid. It's the damage you created in your workout. You sliced and diced your cells. Inflammation comes in to clean up the debris and recruit growth factors to help you rebuild.

If inflammation were Clint Eastwood

Ever seen the movie *The Good, The Bad, and the Ugly*? Inflammation is like one character that can play three different roles. In it's good role, inflammation is like Clint Eastwood, making things temporarily messy for your body in order to restore order to it. In its bad and ugly role, inflammation is like the bad and ugly characters who repeatedly insult and injure your body. In the movie, Clint Eastwood kills the bad and the ugly. In real life, chronic illness will kill you figuratively and literally.

How good inflammation becomes bad and ugly

No matter if inflammation is produced to fight infection or repair a torn bicep, it's all an immune reaction. We've all experienced the acute inflammatory process of red skin and swelling. Short term, acute inflammation is a result of tissue destruction. Chronic inflammation is tissue dysfunction.

Inflammation can be triggered from external events or internal events. External events are things like bacteria, virus, as well as allergens, irritants, toxins, and foreign bodies. Internal events are often from the normal, every day activities of cell turnover that create inflammatory signals. It could be signals from damaged tissue, malfunctioning tissue, and just the normal breakdown of cells. If cells are breaking down faster than programmed, inflammation goes up.

Along those same lines; if you have pain you have inflammation. BUT, you can be inflamed and have no pain. In one third of all heart attacks, the first symptom is death. You can be inflamed and not feel it.

Medications lead to gorilla blindness

Chronic inflammation is like making love to a gorilla. It doesn't stop until the gorilla stops.

Most medications are geared at treating the symptoms of inflammation or cutting out one of the links in the inflammation chain. People may feel better but until they address the underlying reasons that inflammation is being produced, it's going to be a vicious cycle, a.k.a., a Catch 22.

First, drugs suppress symptoms of illness; they do not cure you of illness. So the steroids, antihistamines, and amphetamine-based cold and cough meds you might be taking make you feel better but also allow the little buggers making you sick to stick around longer, keeping you sick longer. Remember, there is a good (not stupid) reason inflammation is being produced.

Second, as the medicine lowers the inflammation response, the body sends MORE inflammatory signals so it can keep up with demand to fight or repair. Your anti-inflammatory medication is actually setting you up to be in a more inflamed state.

Third, the medicine side effects create more damage internally. What happens when damage occurs? Your body activates the immune system to regulate inflammation.

Whether prescription or over-the-counter, NSAIDs (nonsteroidal anti-inflammatory drugs) delay your healing and recovery, and destroy your stomach in the process. A very short list of the generics and brands include ibuprofen (Advil, Motrin), etodalac (Lodine), celecoxib (Celebrex), and aspirin (Bayer, Ascriptin).

If you keep taking the things that keep injuring you, inflammation will have a hard time healing. This is why, in addition to NSAIDs, I caution about the consumption of caffeine, especially after an injury. Caffeine triggers the adrenals, which releases cortisol, which has anti-inflammatory effects on the body by suppressing the immune system. The more caffeine, the longer you deal with the injury.

This is your brain on inflammation...

There are some key players in the inflammation game. The players fall under a broad category of proteins called cytokines (from the Greek cyto for "cell" + kines for "movement").

When you are sick or injured, your immune system cells release cytokines to help protect you. Those proteins may act on the cells they came from, on nearby cells, or on distant cells.

Remember inflammation likes to party. Cytokines can trigger microglial activation. Microglial cells are your first line of defense in your central nervous system (brain and spinal cord). They are the immune cells of your brain.

Remember the purpose of inflammation is to seek and destroy. These microglial cells can destroy the next closest nerve cells, affect neurotransmitter function, or both. The more this happens, the more an auto-immune condition is set up for the brain and mental/emotional conditions.

As a result, MAO (monoamine oxidase) enzyme stimulates the breakdown of the neurotransmitters serotonin and dopamine. Disruptions in these neurotransmitters will affect behavior, mood, memory, concentration, learning, sleep, appetite, and even addiction.

Inflammation can affect the pituitary gland, which disrupts the pathway from brain to adrenals. The more adrenals are fired, the more cortisol is released. The more cortisol is released, the more sugar is dumped into the blood stream. The more sugar is present, the more insulin gets released. But because cortisol is a protective hormone (saves you from a bear) and insulin is a growth hormone (repairs you after the bear attack), cells favor cortisol, and thus insulin resistance ensues.

In short, temporary cortisol is good; constant cortisol is not. Circulating insulin is good; too much circulating insulin is not. You can't be in growth and protection at the same time.

Inflammatory results of obesity

I want to highlight some of the not-so-obvious inflammatory results of being obese. Obesity isn't the only cause of chronic inflammation. I'm highlighting it because of a dilemma: how people perceive beauty versus how people perceive health. You can be big and beautiful; just don't be inflamed and ignorant.

Look around your congregation or organization, how many have weight issues? For the first time in the history of the world, there are more obese people in the us than merely overweight people. Maybe you're one of them.

Ironically, the obesity problem is especially prevalent in the southern states along the Bible belt. I'm sure the Devil loves to see God's people struggle and cry out for prayers. He loves it even more when their prayers aren't answered, proving the lies that God doesn't care about them.

God won't love you any less based on your size. But as a leader, you won't be wrong when you add improved health as a way to worship Him and honor His creation.

If you have excess weight around your butt, gut, and thighs, you have insulin resistance. *But*, just because you are skinny doesn't mean you can't have insulin resistance. I've analyzed many "skinny" people who have elevated A1C (a.k.a. HbA1C) values, elevated fasting insulin levels, or both. I cover these values in more detail in Chapter 12, *Get a Better Blood Panel*. For now, focus on this: *Obesity due to insulin resistance isn't the worst of it.* As noted earlier, some cells are more resistant than others. The endothelial cells—the ones that make up the lining—of your arteries aren't resistant at all. Those cells don't have the genetic capability to become insulin resistant.

So any free-floating insulin that remains in your arteries triggers mitosis: cell division. As the cells lining your arteries start to divide, then your artery walls get thicker, leaving less room for your blood to flow.

Insulin also causes the blood to thicken and turns macrophages (white blood cells) into foam cells. Foam cells are cells that accumulate fatty deposit plaques.

What is a common feature of Alzheimer's and heart disease? Fatty plaques in the brain for Alzheimer's. Fatty plaques in the artery walls for heart disease.

Alzheimer's is now being referred to as Type 3 Diabetes, an insulin resistance of the brain.

To top it off, insulin in high levels is a powerful stimulator of the sympathetic nervous system (protection side), triggering the whole cycle all over again. Even worse, despite your strong spiritual faith and mental care, you can have full blown bear attacks happening internally that you can't feel.

Are those church socials building community that won't

last long since everyone is sick and getting worse? The church isn't the direct cause of its members health problems, but if the church is going to reach more people, they have to offer what people want but don't have. In this case, it can be a culture of health (a judgment free culture of course). Let's serve Jesus more effectively by being able to pour into others more than having to pour into ourselves.

Butt, gut, and thighs: The 24 hour fat store

One of the least resistant areas in the body to store excess energy is that area in the butt, gut, and thighs. We're back to packing on adipose tissue, which releases more cytokines (proteins), which promote C-reactive protein (CRP), and the cycle is happening all over again.

The list of conditions that are affected by inflammation can go on for days. One of the largest areas of inflammation in the body is excessive body fat. Toxins love fatty tissue. The more we are exposed to toxins, the more it's apt to be deposited in fatty tissues. The toxic burden can add to the cytokine load and add more inflammatory insult to inflammatory injury.

Inflammation prevents weight loss

Please hear me when I say this. You can be flabby in the belly but still tight with God. But it's not possible to be healthy and it has nothing to do with you carrying extra weight. It's what those cells produce that lead to volumes of contributing factors for other disease processes.

And also please hear me when I say, it's not about dying

with less weight. There are a thousand ways to lose weight that also don't create health.

But do hear me when I say this. You might be having hard time losing weight because of the amount of inflammation happening. Worry about addressing inflammation and weight loss will be a desired side-effect.

Foods that make your nervous system nervous

Processed foods are the source of so many problems, and three are among the worst: wheat, sugar, and caffeine. They all affect your nervous system in similar ways, so let's use just one, caffeine, as our example.

Caffeine is a drug. It's a legal one but it's still a drug. Because it's a stimulant, caffeine directly affects your adrenals. Your adrenals release two "gas pedal" hormones—adrenaline and cortisol—to help ensure you live another day.

Metabolically, the adrenaline rush increases your cardiac markers: your heart rate, blood pressure, clotting factors, respiratory rate, and cholesterol levels. During stress, a combination of adrenaline and cortisol stimulate emotional and anxiety-inducing memories. Those uncomfortable memories dominate because they help you remember to look for the bear when you're hiking. Too much adrenaline and cortisol too often can be a cause of mental "disorders" or "dis-ease" (as in unease) like depression, anxiety, bipolar behavior, and more.

At the same time that your adrenals are releasing adrenaline and cortisol, your pancreas is releasing a third hormone—insulin—to clean up the aftermath and help move you from protection back to growth.

Short term, the metabolic process for protection will save your life. Long term, it will take your life.

Mind your Ps and foods

Any leader who wants to have an effective and lengthy tenure and still have energy and desire to serve their family, has to take their health seriously. Forget chasing and diagnosing a symptom. This doesn't work.

As you get healthier, your people get healthier. As they get healthier, they have the energy and patience to live out the mission you are preaching. As your flock's energy and passion increases, so does your impact to reach the lost.

With that said, look at your choices of food consumption and run them through the 4 Ps: Philosophy, Purpose, Psychology, and Procedures.

For example, Purpose is your big *why*. So why do you eat a certain way? Is it helping you fuel your mission or helping you fuel your cravings and avoid the next energy crash? I know it's the leadership culture to always show a high energy level, but at some point what goes up must come down.

You can either control the descent or try an Acme parachute. You have to find rest before rest finds you. This is more than just a plea for sleep. If you're using food to keep you going because there's always more to do, the food that gives you sustenance today will be the food that robs you of vitality later.

Your food choices are the easiest habits (Procedures) to change. The calorie in/calorie out notion of health is a farce. You can't exercise your way out of a bad diet. You can't eat your way out of lack of movement. You can't medicate yourself out of chronic illness. And you can't pray your way out of the basic human requirements that are lacking.

How many of your people who plea for prayer requests concerning health crisis are also on medications? They pray for a miracle when in fact God already placed the most amazing ability to heal and repair in their DNA code. They are the miracle. They started as two cells coming together to form one cell and then the miracle of cell division and human development happened.

We all have the blue print for health success; we just have to maintain the blue print with the proper and adequate building materials. Our bodies are temples. Do we want to build and repair the house of God with materials that create more problems?

Remember the Old Testament temple sacrifices were meant to be the first and *best* 10%. Stop offering the leftovers to yourself. It's not serving anyone.

CHAPTER 9

SUGAR, WHEAT, FAT, CHOLESTEROL— FRIENDS OR FOES?

The first part of Romans 12:2 says "Do not be conformed to this world, but be transformed by the renewal of your mind,... ." To me, that verse is a reminder that when you expand your view of certain conditions, you will approach your health strategy differently.

For example, for at least the past 40 years, the media via the government and heart association have drilled the following views into American brains:

- Accept what your doctor says as gospel.

- Follow government recommendations for health initiatives

- Obesity and heart disease are caused by too much fat.

- Cholesterol is an early warning sign of cardio vascular disease (cvd) and other ailments.

- Fat and cholesterol are our enemies.

Attention, steward leaders! It's time to question what's commonly accepted. Let's start with some background about CVD, the attack on fat, and the cholesterol myth.

Cardiovascular disease (CVD)

Every February the media starts its heart disease awareness campaigns. But if you keep following what the media and your doctor push to avoid CVD, you will probably get what most of Americans get: CVD.

The statistics from a 2014 report by the American Heart Association reveals the problem and the contradiction:

- 1 in 3 will die from CVD, which is a death every 40 seconds.

- Every 40 seconds someone has a stroke; and every 4 minutes someone dies from a stroke.

- Deaths have decreased from CVD by 31% from 2000 to 2010.

- There's been a 30% increase in heart related surgeries from 2000 to 2010.

- 920,000 Americans will have a heart attack this year. Half (460,000) will have silent heart attacks.

- Of silent heart attacks, half will have no classic symptoms before or after (such as chest pain); and half will have the mother of all symptoms: they die.

You have people in your congregation who are already part of the statistics. (See Heart disease and stroke statistics--2014 update: a report from the American Heart Association. Circulation. 2014 Jan 21;129(3):e28e292.)

In the spirit of being steward leaders who are taking care of our temporary vessels, I advocate applying a "renew the mind" strategy to healthcare practices by questioning commonly accepted advice, exercising choice, and keeping our 4 Ps aligned. In particular, I hope you renew your mind a bit on the nation's #1 killer, cvd. It's the health issue most likely to take your life and the lives of those you lead. It's also a health issue where, with health courage, you can improve your odds.

A short history of the attack on fat

You can trace the attack on fat to 1976, when Senator George McGovern called a hearing to raise attention about the connection between heart disease and diet.

Eight years later, on March 26, 1984, Time magazine released a cover story showing a plate of two fried eggs and a strip of bacon arranged in a sad face, with the headline *Cholesterol: And Now the Bad News.* The cover story, "Hold the Eggs and Butter," was about the government's longest and most expensive study ever, and started with these words, "Cholesterol is proved deadly, and our diet may never be the same." Americans became obsessed with anything labeled low-fat, and food manufacturers and the media fed the obsession. (See http://time.com/vault/issue/1984-03-26/page/1/ for the cover. For the article, click through to about page 56.)

Twenty-five years later in 2009, the Centers for Disease Control and Prevention (cdc) released its study about obesity.

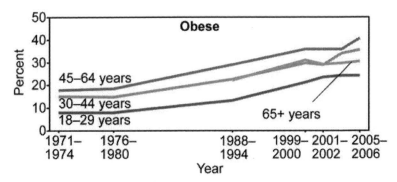

Adapted from "Figure 7. Overweight and Obese," p. 33, *Health, United States, 2008: With Special Feature on the Health of Young Adults.* Source: CDC/NCHS, National Health and Nutrition Examination Survey. National Center for Health Statistics. Hyattsville, MD. 2009. *http://www. cdc.gov/nchs/data/hus/hus08.pdf*

Now there's a contradiction: The 1980s study reported in Time Magazine indicated that high fat diets led to obesity. Given that obesity is among the top three risk factors for heart disease, then shouldn't low fat diets stabilize or decrease obesity rates? Yet the CDC report shows a rise in obesity in a nation obsessed by low-fat foods for more than two decades.

Time magazine smartened up a bit for its June 23, 2014 issue. This time the cover showed an inviting, yellow food swirl with the headline *Eat Butter. Scientists labeled fat the enemy. Why they were wrong.* (See http://time.com/vault/issue/2014-06-23/page/1/ for the cover. For the article, click through to about page 31.)

The origin of the cholesterol myth

The idea of cholesterol as a weapon of mass destruction dates to 1913 when Russian pathologist Nikolai Anitschkow showed that he could produce plaque in the arteries of rabbits by feeding them a diet rich in cholesterol.

Sounds logical, right? It does until you realize rabbits don't eat eggs. Could the damage be occurring because a species was fed something not genetically congruent with their health requirements? Could the same be true for humans today? Are we eating a diet and ingesting medications that are not compatible with our God inspired, innate genetic requirements?

Here's what I want you to know about cholesterol. In protection mode, your body does what it's meant to do to save your life: it raises blood pressure, favors production of LDL over HDL, and dumps sugar into your bloodstream; all so you'll have the heart and leg strength to escape the bear.

Slapping a one-size-fits-all "bad" label on blood pressure and cholesterol is what drives pharmaceutical revenues and results in poor health outcomes.

Sugar and wheat—busted!

I wrote this book in 2016, and 1 in 3 people are still dying of CVD each year.

Maybe it's time to change course. Maybe we should attack sugar intake as this *really can* lead to CVD and other risk factors chased by scientists since the early 1980s.

I'm not talking about the processed sugar carbs alone. Yes, these are contributors but let's attack the "healthy whole grain" carbs and wheat specifically because wheat is a primary source of sugar (a hit on your health) and one of the largest government subsidies (a hit on your wallet).

How dependent on sugar and wheat are you? How pervasive is it in your diet? Why do you care?

Let's start by answering that last question with a brief preview of how your body processes sugar. Then we'll get to the part about how pervasive sugar and wheat are in your diet.

How insulin responds to sugar

In the right forms and amounts, sugar is your friend, not your enemy. Whatever mode you're in, protection or growth, you need sugar to fuel your cells. If your cells aren't getting enough sugar, then your body will literally rip itself apart to obtain it. Otherwise, if there's too much sugar available, it gets stored.

When you consume sugar, your body has an *insulin response* where insulin attempts to store the sugar for later use. Insulin first attempts to store the sugar in the liver and muscles, where the sugar is converted into glycogen. When your cells need energy, the glycogen is converted to glucose.

Your liver and muscles store a limited amount of sugar. Once you fill up your glycogen stores (about an active day's worth), the liver and muscles stop producing glycogen, and the liver starts producing triglycerides (medical-speak for globules of fat). Insulin carries the triglycerides to areas of your body where there's plenty of storage space for it: your butt, gut, and thighs.

Mind the glycemic index and load

Sugar—not fat—triggers an insulin response that leads to the formation of triglycerides. Low fat foods tend to be high sugar foods. When you remove fat, your remove the flavor. For the low fat or fat-free food to taste good, you have to add sugar. Just look at the sugar grams in a serving of a low-fat yogurt.

The *glycemic index* rates how high a food will raise your blood sugar levels. Glucose—the pure form of sugar that your body uses for energy—is the gold standard with a score of 100. Higher glycemic foods are easier to digest, which makes them easier to convert to glucose, which makes it easier to trigger an insulin response. Here are a few examples of foods and their glycemic indexes:

Glycemic Index of Common Foods

High: 70-100+		Medium: 56-69		Low: 0-55	
Baked russet potato	111	White basmati	67	Oatmeal	55
Fruit Roll Ups	99	Raisins	64	Quinoa	53
Baguette	95	Banana	62	Snickers	51
White rice	89	Honey	61	Brown rice	50
Pretzels	83	Sweet corn on the cob	60	Vanilla cake from mix with vanilla frosting	42
Gatorade	78	Grapes	59	Orange	40
Grape nuts	75	Ice cream	57	Apple	39
Graham crackers	74			Pear	38
Wonder Bread	73			M & M's, peanut	33
Bagel	72			Black beans	30
Whole wheat bread	71			Cashews	27

Adapted from "Glycemic index and glycemic load for 100+ foods" at http://www.health.harvard.edu/diseases-and-conditions/glycemic_index_and_glycemic_load_for_100_foods.

As you study the list, notice how many are low fat, high-carb, and wheat-based, like bagels, pretzels, and graham crackers. Ever wonder why eating low fat isn't budging the fat or is even making you fat? Look to the processed-wheat products. Pretzels have a higher glycemic index (83) than a serving of frosted vanilla cake (42) with a side of M&Ms (33).

Don't be misled, however, into thinking "Great! I'd rather have vanilla cake than a bagel anyway!" Because in addition to the glycemic index, you need to consider the glycemic *load*, a measure of how many carbs you are consuming.

Though it may have a lower sugar spike compared to a bagel, the vanilla cake pretty much packs the same amount of carbs per 10 grams of serving: 25 for the bagel and 24 for the vanilla cake. (To see the numbers for yourself, go to the Harvard link cited in the glycemic index table.)

I've seen countless triathletes and distance runners with flabby bellies because they carb load so much. They get their exercise on, depleting the glycogen stores in their liver and muscles. Knowing that they're supposed to eat something after exercise, they reach for the low fat pretzels. This is also why so many people have trouble losing weight; they think the low-fat pretzels = less body fat.

The truth is, your body will use the easy-to-get sugar before the hard-to-get sugar. Foods with high glycemic indexes and glycemic loads, like pretzels, are easy sugar. Those pretzels are rapidly turned into glucose that goes right back into the muscles and liver. When your muscles and liver are sugar-satiated, the excess sugar gets shipped to the fat stores (your butt, gut, and thighs), a process that that jacks up triglycerides (sugar attached to fat), glycosylated proteins like

A1C (sugar attached to protein), and insulin production.

Ultimately you want to consume and eat foods that have a lower glycemic index so you can regulate your insulin response better. With that said, don't be afraid of all carbs. Just be afraid of the ones that have a high glycemic index, and most importantly, ones that have both a high glycemic index and glycemic load. This is why you can't go wrong with fruits and veggies as snacks and a main stay in your diet. I'll talk more about this in Part III, *Your 7 Day Jump Start to Health.*

How sugar AGEs you and cholesterol helps you

Your body is always in a state of adaptation and won't leave you with high blood sugar. In an attempt to diminish the damaging effects of blood sugar, your body will combine the sugar onto a protein, creating advanced glycosylated end products (AGES).

The AGES make your cells stiffer, less pliable, and more susceptible to damage and rapid aging. If cells are being damaged and aging faster, this is a recipe for oxidation and inflammation. Think of the process like burning toast; you cannot "un-toast" bread. Once an AGE is formed, it's irreversible. To get rid of it, the body attacks it. Attacking = inflammation.

Therein lies the good news/bad news...inflammation. If you get a cut, your skin swells up (inflammation). Cholesterol rushes to the scene to patch it up. You form a scab and unless you keep ripping the scab off, your body heals nicely.

But if that wound is in your arteries (from sugar and AGES), where you don't feel it, cholesterol is rushed to the scene by LDL and VLDL to patch it up. Since it's an injury, inflammation occurs to aid in the repair. You form a scab (plaque) in the artery like you just did on your skin.

In this case, since your AGES are elevated, it's like repeatedly ripping off the scab as well as creating new cuts for your body to repair. Due to swelling and scabs forming on top of scabs, the diameter of the artery diminishes.

What gets blamed? Cholesterol. You've seen it 1,000 times. It's never the kid who instigates the fight that gets caught, it's the one who reacts. Cholesterol is reacting to too much sugar. AGES and inflammation are the instigators.

Rewind the video to see how the fight actually started. I'm sure you'll see a lot of sugar involved in the form of wheat, sugar, and the effects of caffeine.

CHAPTER 10

CORTISOL, INSULIN, AND YOUR IMMUNE SYSTEM

Cortisol is your sugar dumper

Adrenaline and cortisol are the major hormones released by your adrenals. The prime role of cortisol is to dump sugar into the blood stream so you have instant energy to escape the bear.

Most people in the health and leadership industries look at cortisol as a stress hormone. It's not a stress hormone, it's a *survival* hormone. Remember, the body will favor survival over sex, life over legacy, protection over growth...every time.

Whereas cortisol is a hormone that protects us by dumping sugar into our blood so we have enough energy to outrun the bear, insulin protects us by taking excess sugar out of our blood so we don't go into coma from a sugar overdose.

Insulin is your sugar distributor

Insulin is a growth hormone with many roles. It aids virtually every cell function—including cell division—by delivering sugar (glucose) and other nutrients to cells.

The better your body responds to insulin, then the easier it is for you to lose weight, gain energy, to recover from illness, and to inhibit cancer and other types of diseases. But when your body is confused about its insulin needs, diabetes and other chronic illnesses show up.

God made humans in His image and we are wonderfully made. Our bodies don't do stupid things. We do. Like confusing our bodies about its insulin needs.

If you have a breakfast of a coffee, donut, and cereal (caffeine, sugar, and wheat), then your blood sugars are being signaled to rev up for anything that may attack you.

It's a good thing that God is in charge because he also created our body to help regulate that excess blood sugar, a.k.a. insulin response. The process works like this:

1. Insulin first transports sugar (glucose) to your muscles and liver.

2. When your muscles and liver get their fill (about a day's worth of energy), then the excess sugar attaches to fat, wherever it can find the fat, in the form of triglycerides (globules of fat).

3. Insulin transports the triglycerides to your body's fat storehouses, (your butt, gut, and thighs are the biggest storehouses).

Here's the bottom-line: control insulin, control your health. In addition to eating a low-glycemic diet, sleep is one of the best ways to control insulin.

Your two-armed immune system

When your nervous system is stuck in protection mode, what happens to your immune system? It gets whacked, too.

For simplicity, your immune system has two arms. One arm is the side that promotes inflammation like the runny nose, fever, vomiting and diarrhea; signs that the threat to your body is being contained so it can't spread. The other arm is the antibody side that neutralizes the threat and recruit other cells or proteins to kill it so body can heal. For a fully functioning immune system, you need both arms working together, in conjunction.

Say you're running from a bear. You jump over a log and twist your ankle. You think, "This is it. The bear will get me, I won't be able to run anymore."

You inspect your ankle for damage; you can move it around, you can put pressure on it, and it's only slightly swollen. You get back on your feet and keep running though it may be a little stiff and painful.

After 20 minutes of running, you're safe. You collapse in exhaustion. When you try to get up, you collapse again. You look at your ankle; it's now ballooned and hanging over your shoe top. It's *painful* and looks like you may have to cut your shoe off.

It wouldn't be conducive to blow up your ankle when you have a bear chasing you. Now that you're safe, the protection side can fire less and the growth side takes over to aid in repair and growth.

Or think of it like your college days. You cram the final

two weeks of the semester studying. Energy is high, you feel good, but as soon as you get home for Christmas break, you crash. You wake up the next day with a runny nose, coughing, and sweating bullets.

You blame it on "catching a bug" when you got home. In reality, you were sick while cramming but because you were in protection mode, your nervous system told your immune system to chill until you're safe.

CHAPTER 11

THE 5 PILLARS OF ILLNESS YOU NEED TO CONQUER

God created our nervous systems to tell our bodies when to be in protection and survival mode or growth and repair mode. Though He made our bodies to favor survival over growth, God never intended our bodies to always be in one mode or the other.

Chronic illness is a sign that your body's nervous system is *stuck* in protection or, worse, totally burned out.

To understand how your nervous system can get stuck in protection mode, imagine illness as five interacting pillars:

1. Autonomic imbalance
2. Adrenal dysfunction
3. Insulin resistance
4. Immune dysfunction
5. Chronic inflammation

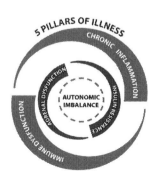

A trigger in one pillar can trigger a cascade in the other pillars. Although the cascade isn't necessarily sequential, over time, it becomes a vicious cycle that keeps your nervous system in protection mode. Your gas pedal is always floored.

Before tackling how to break the cycle, let's look at how each of the pillars contribute to chronic illness.

1. Autonomic imbalance

Your nervous system sets the stage for coordinating and organizing your life into protection or growth mode. Look at your protection side like your car's gas pedal, and your growth side like your brake pedal.

You cannot be in growth and protection mode at the same time. An autonomic imbalance means that you've been operating in one mode—typically protection—for too long. And that puts you at an increased risk of disease and ailments.

If you are always on the gas pedal, the only way to stop is to run out of gas or to crash. Neither is a successful outcome.

Being on a brake pedal constantly makes the brakes smoke and burn out. Your only line of defense is to cry when the bill comes due for a new set of brakes.

2. Adrenal dysfunction

Cortisol is a protection hormone. It floods your body with sugar to give you the energy to outrun whatever is trying to hurt or kill you.

When your body is over-producing cortisol, then it's dumping sugar too much and too often which leads to illnesses such as thyroid dysfunction, hormone dysregulation, and cognitive impairments. Too much cortisol also sets you up for the other pillars of illness: insulin resistance, chronic inflammation, immune dysfunction, and autonomic imbalance.

3. Insulin resistance

Insulin resistance is a term you hear thrown around a lot in reference to diabetes and obesity. Let's say you have a breakfast of a Frappuccino, a bagel, and a diet Coke (you're watching your calories after all). That's a hurricane of sugar rushing into your blood stream. To make sure your body doesn't go into a coma, the pancreas releases insulin hormones to escort the sugar into your cells. In other words, you're storing energy for later.

Your cells are very sensitive and get annoyed easily. Too much insulin irritates them and they stop listening. Put another way, your cells are the mom, and insulin is the toddler. The toddler keeps tapping on mom's arm while repeatedly saying, "Mom, mom, mom, mom, mom... ." The mom, trying to have a conversation with her friend, starts ignoring the toddler's pleas. So the toddler has to yell louder to get mom's attention. It's only a matter of time before mom (your cells) becomes deaf to toddler (insulin) pleas for attention.

Consequently, the sugar doesn't get stored in cells and blood sugar rises while your body figures out which of two storage routes to use to deal with the excess sugar. The first is to combine the sugar with three fatty acids to form triglycerides, which are then formed into saturated fat and easily deposited in your midsection. The second route is attaching sugar to a protein, like hemoglobin, a protein found in your red blood cells. I cover why this is very damaging to your body and why you don't want to rely on "normal" test values in Chapter 12, but for now, drill this into your head: It's absurd to attack fat as the reason for obesity and heart disease. Fat is not the problem. *Sugar is the problem.* One of the best strategies at reversing your heart problems, obesity, diabetes, or what ails you is to consume a higher fat diet (more about that in Chapter 13).

By now you "get" that insulin is a growth hormone with the role of storing sugar and nutrients. Here's something you might not know: insulin is also a *mitogenic* hormone. This means insulin stimulates cell division. In other words, cells are replicating faster than programmed. Cells dividing more rapidly is what we call aging but also the basis of every known cancer. When we become insulin resistant, the risk factors for breast cancer, ovarian cancer, endometriosis, PCOS, prostate cancer, heart disease, diabetes, obesity, and even Alzheimer's and dementia skyrocket.

The first place insulin resistance happens is in the liver and then in the muscles. The last place is the butt, gut, and thighs. The latest cognitive impairment research is calling brain degenerative diseases like Parkinson's, Alzheimer's, and dementia Type 3 diabetes because it's an insulin resistance problem in the brain. So when you hear brain ailments, start thinking insulin resistance.

4. Immune system dysfunction

When you have an autonomic imbalance, your immune system takes a back seat to protection. Because 70-80% of your immune system resides in the gut, poor immune health is also poor gut health.

Poor gut health can result in conditions like poor digestion (usually a lack of stomach acid), or poor elimination,
either of which can create leaky gut: holes in your intestines.
Proteins that should stay in your gut escape into your blood
stream and other parts of your body.

The body attacks the proteins that don't belong in the
"hood," and builds antibodies to neutralize them. Those antibodies can then attack other tissues while continuing to look
for the enemy. That creates more inflammation which can
trigger the protection cycle, over and over.

5. Chronic inflammation

When you have chronic inflammation, your body never heals.
Your body constantly trying to adapt to survive is one source
of inflammation. The more adaptation your body has to do
to survive, the more inflammation you'll experience, and the
more likely you'll suffer from disease. Many will say chronic
inflammation is the root cause of disease; but I assert that
poor lifestyle choices are the root cause. Here's why: poor
choices lead to deficiency and toxicity, which leads to chronic
inflammation, which leads to disease.

Another source of inflammation is free-radical production. Increased energy expenditure creates more free radical
byproducts. Free radicals rip apart tissues and even your
DNA. As you influence your DNA expression, you influence your
health and life expression.

CHAPTER 12

GET A BETTER BLOOD PANEL

A lot of my day is spent analyzing lab work. Most people will visit their doctor; get that "standard-of-care" blood panel, and be told everything looks good based on the normal reference ranges.

Why your standard blood panel is substandard

There are several problems with your standard blood panel, making it a substandard test for identifying the root causes of problems. The normal reference ranges lump 95% of the American population as normal and healthy. Look at 95% of your congregation. Would you call them healthy? The mere fact that 80% of healthcare claims are for chronic illness should put a glaring point to everyone that it's impossible to call 95% of the population healthy and normal.

The information you can glean from the standard-of-care reference ranges is very limited. It may catch something if you are grossly out of range but leaves too much of a grey area in your health story. This is why I tighten up the ranges when analyzing labs. Tighter ranges help create a clearer picture of everything and allows me to focus on systems over symptoms, and origins over organs.

Don't chase the hormones

One trap I'm seeing more and more of is testing for hormones. Guys want to know their testosterone values and women want to know their estrogen/progesterone balance.

Here's one thing to consider before seeking treatment for hormone deficiencies. Hormone production is dependent on the nervous system. If you are operating out of the protection side of life more often than not, you will not produce growth hormones like you desire. You can't be in growth and protection at the same time.

Another fun fact is that cholesterol is the basis of many hormones but is a limited resource. If you are facing a bear, you body will shunt cholesterol into the production of cortisol before it offers these valuable building blocks to formulate estrogen and progesterone and testosterone.

Hormone imbalances are an effect of deficiency and toxicity; the skid marks at the scene of an accident.

The labs you should be getting but aren't

You should badger your doctor into including a few more analytes—doctorspeak for substances of interest—on your next labs:

1. A1C a.k.a. HbA1C a.k.a. Hemoglobin A1C

2. CRP (C-reactive protein)

3. Homocysteine

4. Vitamin D (25–Hydroxy)

5. Fasting insulin

For a summary understanding of these analytes and why testing is important, keep reading. For even more information, go to http://www.morehealthlesshealthcare.com/lab-values/biomarkers-that-mean-something/

A1C test (a.k.a. HbA1C a.k.a. hemoglobin test)

Hemoglobin is a protein found in your red blood cells. When sugar attaches itself to hemoglobin, the result is A1C, the super-short name for glycosylated hemoglobin.

Purpose. This is the 3-4 month average of your blood sugars. The test is used to measure the amount of sugar attached to hemoglobin. Hemoglobin is the oxygen-carrying component of your red blood cells.

Red blood cells live about 90-120 days so an A1C test can give you an estimated 3-4 months blood sugar average, volumes more accurate than a fasting blood glucose test.

Why it's important. A1C is more than a marker for sugar utilization; the value of this test goes way beyond if you're "pre-diabetic." First, your body may decide that it has more excess sugar than your fat cells can handle, so it next looks for storage capacity in proteins like hemoglobin. Second, remember that when sugar binds to proteins it results in AGES, and AGES rip apart your body (see the earlier topic, "How sugar AGES you and cholesterol helps you"). I use an A1C test to flag if excess sugar is being stored in hemoglobin, and if so to assess how much damage is occurring. The more damage, the more inflammation. The more inflammation, the less quality and quantity of health and life.

Frequency. If it's outside the optimal range, then test two to three times a year; otherwise, test once or twice a year.

Problem with normal. The "normal" ranges are 4.8-5.6% as healthy; 5.7%-6.4% as pre-diabetic, and >6.4% as diabetic.

Values I flag. I get nervous when I see levels under 4.7% or over 5.4%.

Elevated numbers may indicate. The higher your A1C, the more stress and damage is occurring in the body. There are exceptions, but in general, an elevated number is a good starting point to quantify damage.

Low to moderate numbers may indicate. A persistently low A1C is a red flag for chronic problems like hypoglycemia, adrenal insufficiency, anemia, and antioxidant insufficiencies. Reduced numbers over time are a good starting point to quantify if you are improving and if you are preventing excessive damage.

CRP (C-reactive protein) test

Recall that inflammation is a helper that, under normal circumstances, does its job and then goes away. Cytokines are the messengers used by the immune system to trigger help. CRP is a protein produced in the liver in response to the cytokines; i.e., CRP is a signal, if you will, that inflammation is occurring.

Purpose. The test can be used to help assess cardiac risk as well as chronic and systemic problems. It's a very sensitive marker for the presence of inflammation but not its cause.

Why it's important. A CRP test is a great tool for detecting inflammation and monitoring health improvement. Any chronic elevation should be treated and managed.

Problem with normal. Because there is no safe limit for CRP, there is no "normal" range to flag.

Frequency. Test regularly.

Values I flag. In today's toxic and deficient world, I expect to see elevated CRP. Given that 0.0 mg/L is ideal, my buffer is <0.5 mg/L; if the number is over that, then I want to investigate the reasons.

Elevated numbers may indicate. Elevations over 7.0 mg/L are more likely due to acute infections and trauma. CRP is not elevated in *all* causes of inflammation. An IUD (intra-uterine device) works by causing inflammation in the uterus and may elevate CRP levels.

Low to moderate numbers may indicate. At 0.5–7.0 mg/L, inflammation is more likely due to chronic and systemic conditions like heart disease, as well as autoimmune disorders such as rheumatoid arthritis, neurological disorders such as epilepsy, and GI (gastro-intestinal) problems.

Notes. CRP attaches to cell membranes to attract immune cells for clean up. The catch is that CRP is released in response to other inflammatory signals but has the ability to signal for more. For example, fat cells produce the IL-6 protein, which tells the liver to produce more CRP, and CRP produces inflammation all over. Inflammation likes to party and signals for the master of ceremonies, NFkB. In other words, I don't look at obesity as a fat problem; I look at it as an *inflammatory* problem.

For a deep understanding of NFKB, read *Grain Brain* by David Perlmutter, MD, a book I recommend to many of my clients.

Homocysteine test

Amino acids are the building blocks of proteins. You can get some of your amino acids from diet, but others need to be produced by your body. Homocysteine is an amino acid that your body produces when you consume meat, fish, or dairy.

Purpose. The homocysteine test is used to assess your risk for over 100 disorders (hormone imbalances, autoimmune problems, mental problems, and more) that will shorten your life and decrease your quality of life.

Why it's important. Homocysteine is often called the single best indicator of your longevity and quality of life because too much of it is both an indicator of disease and a massive contributor to it. It's a contributor to disease because it damages the linings of your arteries.

Frequency. If numbers are elevated, test 3-4 times/year.

Problem with normal. Your traditional lab value won't flag a problem until you're over 15 umol/L, when it's too late to take preventive action.

Values I flag. I like to see a homocysteine range between 4-8 umol/L.

Elevated numbers may indicate. A number >8 umol/L is enough to get me antsy. Too much homocysteine can lead to cardio vascular disease, Alzheimer's, Parkinson's, diabetes hypothyroidism, osteoporosis, autism, anemia, and other disorders.

Low to moderate numbers may indicate. A number <4umol/L may indicate malnourishment or malabsorption problems, antioxidant deficiencies, hyperthyroidism, medication use (antibiotics, birth control, and tamoxifen to name a few), liver disease, and kidney disease. Notice the list included medication. That's because just because it's prescribed does not mean it's safe.

Vitamin D (25–Hydroxy)

Though often categorized as a vitamin, vitamin D is actually a hormone. Most vitamins cannot be produced by the cells in your body and must be obtained from dietary sources. Vitamin D is an exception: It can be made by the cells in your body by converting cholesterol derivatives into vitamin D using sunlight. (Yet another example of why cholesterol, as God intended it, is a good thing.)

The "25 hydroxy" in the test name refers to the second conversion stage when vitamin D3 is converted to D25hydroxy (the one we mostly test for) in your liver. Here's a quick look at the conversion process:

1. Your skin absorbs ultraviolet B light (uvʙ) from the sun.

2. Your skin cells produce D3 (a.k.a. cholecalciferol) which then goes to your liver.

3. Your liver converts D3 to D25-hydroxylase (a.k.a. 25hydroxycholecalciferol), which then goes to your kidneys.

4. In your kidneys, D25-hydroxylase is converted to a biologically active vitamin: D1,25-hydroxy, (a.k.a. calcitriol a.k.a. D1,25-hydroxycholecalciferol).

Purpose. The test is used primarily to assess if you are getting enough vitamin D. Being sufficient in vitamin D is essential for wellness and disease prevention. Being deficient can lead to increased risk of many otherwise-preventable diseases.

Why it's important. Many cells have vitamin D receptors and many genes are influenced by the action of vitamin D. In fact, it's been estimated that the human genome has over 2,700 binding sites for vitamin D. That's why biologically active vitamin D is often considered the most potent steroid hormone in human physiology. With so much of your body relying on vitamin D, testing is the only way to know if you are getting the right amount.

Frequency. Test 3-4 times/year until numbers are >50 ng/ml; then test 1-2 times/year.

Problem with normal. Typical lab ranges will have an ocean of normal between 30-100 ng/ml. You can have a value of 30.1 and they say you're okay because you are a mere step above preventing rickets.

Values I flag. The Vitamin D Council (www.vitamindcouncil.org) suggests a level of 50 ng/ml. I want to be proactive, so I favor a value between 50-90 ng/ml.

Elevated numbers may indicate. Though difficult to get too much vitamin D, it can happen. Not from sunlight or foods, but from taking high does of supplements for too long.

A number over 90 ng/ml is my trigger to look for elevated blood calcium, which could be the cause of nausea, constipation, confusion, abnormal heart rhythm, and kidney stones.

Low to moderate numbers may indicate. When there is any deficiency in Vitamin D, this can lead to a disruption in virtually any function of the body. But know this: If you are deficient, it doesn't always mean that you have a lack of consumption or a lack of sun exposure. Those vitamin D compounds have to be chemically altered through the liver and kidneys to become active. So deficiencies could mean that you have to look deeper at a dysfunctional liver or kidney. So keep this mind: the fastest way to trash your liver and kidneys is by creating an internal environment of insulin resistance as well as consuming painkiller and pharmaceutical anti-inflammatories.

Fasting Insulin

If you can control insulin, you can control lifespan and quality of life. There isn't an illness that doesn't have roots in poor insulin regulation. Anything from obesity, diabetes, heart disease, Alzheimer's, autism, degenerative disc disease, chronic pain, pcos, breast cancer, restless leg syndrome, chronic fatigue, osteoporosis, fatty liver disease, thyroid disorders, high cholesterol, and hypertension.

Purpose. The test measures how much insulin is circulating in your body, especially when you haven't eaten.

Why it's important. Why would you want a fasting insulin if you already have good levels of A1C and glucose? Because your pancreas may be working overtime to make sure those other values (A1C and glucose) are fine. Your pancreas can only keep up for so long before burnout. A fasting insulin gives context to how hard your body is working to maintain your sugar load.

Frequency. Test quarterly until your insulin is stabilized, then test 1-2 times/year.

Problem with normal. Lab A might report you have a problem at 8 mIU/L, while Lab B reports "you're all good" for anything lower than 25 mIU/L. Waiting until your fasting insulin is 25 before taking action is like waiting until you're 84 years old to start saving for retirement. You need to start praying for miracles.

Values I flag. For fasting insulin, I want to see a range of 2-5 mIU/L, with 3 ideal. These are the same values recommended by Dr. David Perlmutter, the author of *Grain Brain* (a book mentioned earlier in "C-reactive protein test").

Elevated numbers may indicate. A number >5 mIU/L may indicate you are producing too much insulin, a contributor to obesity and eventually to producing insufficient insulin because your pancreas can't keep up.

Low to moderate numbers may indicate. A number below 2 mIU/L is a concern because it indicates either you've burned out your pancreas or you have an autoimmune condition that doesn't allow your pancreas to produce enough insulin.

Labs have you curious?

Blood panel labs are an important tool in your healthcare

toolkit. The information in your labs can help you with healthy decision making, *if* you're getting the right information. It's your health; don't settle for the customary "standard of care panel" that does little but shift you into being a life long customer for statins and other drugs.

Taking action now means you're less likely to need miracles later. If you want to know your CRP, homocysteine, A1C, vitamin D, and fasting insulin and ways to optimize those values to optimize your health expression, you know how to find me.

CHAPTER 13

WHAT TO EAT

Make friends with fat

One of the best ways to build up your brake pedal is to build up your fat intake. Don't be afraid of fat. Fat is your friend. If you have excess body fat or if you've had the lab tests just described in Chapter 12 and your results are abnormal, then I recommend getting jiggy with fatty foods.

You may fear that I'm going to put you on a rabbit food diet and more calorie restriction. Instead, I want you to get ketogenic, which means you are burning fat as fuel, not sugar. To do that, you'll need to start eating fat and *stop* eating sugar. Easier said than done, I know; not eating sugar can be difficult. According to research by Dr. David Ludwig, M.D., Ph.D., when the brain is exposed to sugar, then the part of the brain that lights up is the very same part that is triggered by cocaine or heroin. He also states that there are 600,000 food items in America and 80% of them have added sugar.

Needless to say, your battle begins with your points of purchase, but also by retraining your brain. Start with two easy lessons.

Lesson #1: Fat is flavor. When fat is removed so is flavor. So manufacturers have to add sugar to make low-fat and no-fat foods palatable.

Lesson #2. To skip the sugar, enjoy the fat. Here's a short list what you should be eating:

- eggs
- bacon
- sausage
- beef
- chicken
- fish
- wild game
- more eggs
- avocados
- olives
- seeds and nuts
- seed and nut butters
- coconut butter

I know some of you are going to have your panties in a tizzy over pork products. If that's you, don't eat pork. If it's not you, don't worry about it. Eating pork products may violate your ethics but it's not going to violate your salvation.

The cleaner the source, the better, which means avoiding hormones and antibiotic-filled meats.

Eating more fat is probably the opposite advice you are getting from your traditional doctor or trainer. I'm sure if you pass this information along to your followers, you will get people looking at you as if you're a crazy person. They want you on a low fat diet, which means a high sugar diet.

A side note: Don't make this into an Atkins diet where the only thing you do eat is meat. Remember I said veggies and fruits? Don't forget that part. It was the Garden of Eden, not the Pasture of Eden.

Fat is like a savings account. If we have money coming in, we are more likely to spend money. When we don't have money coming in, we are more likely to hold onto money. I'm sure your ministry has gone through these ebbs and flows. Tithes or revenue was down so you tightened up the budget

WHAT TO EAT? **139**

or maybe even had to cut ties with programs and support people. The body isn't much different.

When our body sees fat coming in, our body relaxes on storing it and we lose weight. When we don't ever have fat coming in, our body holds onto it, creating weight loss frustration. But again, it's not just about weight loss; that's just a desired side effect for many people.

Side note. For more information about how manufacturers seduce our taste buds by adding sodium, sweeteners, and unnatural fats to food, read the book *Salt, Sugar, Fat: How the Food Giants Hooked Us,* by Michael Moss. The title says it all.

What should you drink?

Water, water, and water. I want you to shoot for ½ your weight in ounces each day. The type of water is not that important, with one exception: *no* tap water. Tap water is filled with industrial chemicals, pharmaceuticals, and hormones that other people pee out when their bodies don't utilize them. (You'll learn more about water in Part III, on Day 1 of *Your 7 Day Jump Start to Health.*)

Juices (natural or not), soda, milk, coffee, and alcohol will all sky rocket your blood sugars. Milk may have a low glycemic value but it has a high insulin response. In effect, it has the same response in the body as bread. The nation of Israel was looking for the Land of Milk and Honey. It's here, and if you only consume milk and honey, there's a good chance you'll meet your Maker sooner than later.

What about snacks?

Does it contain high fat content? Go for it. Does it contain high sugar content? Avoid it like the plague. When in doubt, don't eat anything. Your body knows what to do better in an underfed state than in an over fed state. Protein shakes are great for snacks. Again, make sure they aren't filled with garbage like colors, sweeteners, artificial flavors, or ingredients you can't pronounce.

Raw rules

Raw fruits and veggies are amazing for you in every aspect, especially helping to build and maintain a healthy immune system. Here are a few of the benefits. Raw produce:

- Contains nutrients, phytonutrients, enzymes, co-enzymes, and fiber, and countless antioxidants that help fight free-radical production.

- Alkalizes the blood, which makes hydrogen more prevalent, and hydrogen beats the crap out of cancer cells.

- Contains countless antioxidants. Antioxidants fight free radical production..., which beats the crap out of cancer.

Fasting

You may know an underfed state as "fasting." Jesus did it for a while. Moses did it for awhile. Not only can fasting clear your belly of blood sugar crashing foods, it can clear your mind for deeper thought and emotional connection with God as you prepare your sermons.

One thing I admire about my pastor, Kelly Williams of

Vanguard Church, is that he fasts the days he writes his sermons. But don't do it because someone else does it because that's the hard way.

The easy way is to understand your own *why* for fasting; then your *do* will be easier and lasting. And when you're doing it, don't over-do it. Fasting for too long or too often can have detrimental effects, especially if you are not already healthy. I often start people who are new to fasting with 12 hours each day, which is pretty easy to accomplish. Just measure the hours from the last meal at night until first meal of the next day.

CHAPTER 14

MOVEMENT IS THE NEW NUTRIENT

As much as we're told to move and exercise more, the real problem is we're too sedentary. Someone who vigorously exercises for two hours a day and spends the other twenty two mostly sitting and sleeping is sedentary.

If you believe the statistics—the average American sits 60% of the day, and 8-18 year olds are closer to 80% sedentary—then it's not hard to visualize a nation of Jabba the Hutt contenders.

Because it's not a substance, some would argue movement couldn't possibly be a nutrient. But I assert that movement is a nutrient as essential to your health as minerals, proteins, fats, carbohydrates, and water.

Here's why: an inadequate amount of any nutrient is a deficiency, and you need movement to help ensure that (1) other nutrients are absorbed, recycled, and excreted as they should be, and (2) your cerebellum isn't bypassed when you need it most.

Sitting is the new smoking

The effects of movement on your cerebellum may not be obvious, so here's the short explanation. In your biology class, you were probably taught that your cerebellum controlled your balance, coordination, and other motor skills. In fact, your cerebellum also works with other parts of your brain to coordinate your thoughts and memories, learning, and emotions, and to reduce stress.

Movement signals your nervous system to tell your cerebellum to do its job. Your nervous system interprets sitting as lack of movement, and when you sit too long your nervous system bypasses your cerebellum and heads towards your cortex (possibly giving you a headache) or your adrenals (making you anxious and on bear alert).

Headaches and anxiety may be minor problems compared to the dangers of prolonged sitting. Too much sitting starves your brain, and a starved brain is not patient or present with people. A starved brain leads to diagnoses of some disorder that gets treated with medications that alter the brain even more.

Even if you work out regularly, sitting all day shifts you away from growth and repair into survival and protection. Prolonged sitting is tied to an increased risk of diabetes, obesity, heart disease, liver disease, metabolic syndrome, and early death.

Becoming a standup steward leader

Obviously I want you to exercise; more importantly, I want you to *not* be sedentary by standing more. It takes over 200 muscles to stand still and not fall over. Standing is not vigorous but it is strenuous. Strenuous is good for you.

You may need to ease into standing. You might at first want to alternate your chair with an exercise ball. If you don't have knee problems, you could also kneel on a yoga block (one knee at a time) while working at a traditional height desk. Switch knees every 5-10 minutes.

Eventually I want you to change your work-station. Instead of a traditional desk and chair, I want you to create or buy a desk that you use while standing.

Increment these changes slowly. Start with 10% of your day on the exercise ball or yoga block. When that feels fine, increase your time to 20%. Then work towards a goal where you spend 85% or more of your day standing while at your workstation.

You may feel a little achy for the first week or two each time you increase your standing. This is expected and normal.

It took me about a year to transition from mostly sitting to mostly standing. Now I have a standing-only work station. I built it out of a closet organizer from Lowes. I can add shelving and more space as needed. I'm also not meeting with clients in my office so it doesn't have to look pretty. I've written this entire book while standing.

My assistant stands at the front desk. She doesn't have a chair. She would complain if I made her sit.

Because of the physical demand of standing all day, you'll be tired at night, ready to hit the bed at a good hour, and you'll sleep better. The more restful your sleep, the better the repair and recovery of your body from the day's stressors.

Why do you deliver a sermon or keynote standing? Why not stand to do your other work, giving it the same confidence-building intent and attention as you do on a Sunday morning?

Is cardio hurting more than helping?

Even though exercise is beneficial, it's a stress because it shifts your body into protection mode. Your body will react the same way whether you're doing a pull-up or pulling yourself up a fence to escape an angry dog.

The longer your workout the more you place your body into protection mode. If your body is already firing in protection, then adding long, drawn-out cardio sessions (especially with little variation) can harm more than help. Exercise is the least effective tool to lose weight. Instead, you need exercise to feed your brain and nervous system.

Remember, in protection mode your adrenals release cortisol and this dumps sugar into your blood. At the same time, your pancreas releases insulin to collect excess sugar to make sure you don't go into a diabetic coma.

Insulin will transport excess sugar first to your liver and muscles, leaving enough to give you about a day's worth of stored energy. If there's still some left, insulin transports the remaining sugar to your belly, butt, thighs and other storehouses where the sugar is converted to fat and kept as backup energy.

When the sugar in your liver and muscles is depleted—

and your body cannot get sugar any other way—*then* the fat gets attention. It doesn't matter what kind of exercise you are doing, the order your body uses sugar is the same. But here's the critical difference: When cardio exercise stops, so does sugar burning. When lean muscle building exercise stops, sugar burning continues, even during periods of inactivity, including sleep.

How do you build lean muscle? You have to push and pull things; climb on and jump over things; and fall down and get up, and sprint. You have to do the things that will help you be fit enough to fight and escape bears.

Your fitness level is directly proportional to your survival and protection level. By fitness, I mean your body's ability to adapt to changing situations. If you're always on a treadmill, elliptical, or stationary bike, how does that serve your ability to adapt? It's the same pace and the same distance every time. That's why I'm not a fan of long cardio sessions, unless you're training for a marathon or distance race.

Think back to the bear attack. How would you survive the bear? Would you keep a nice steady pace? Only if you want to be eaten. More likely, you would sprint, jump, and climb. So create a fitness routine around movements that could help you survive a bear attack.

Should bear attacks not resonate with you, then try looking at it another way. If you fell down, how fast could you get up? If you had to protect your child from something, could you lift him or her and jump, sprint, or climb to safety?

Remember, your ability to adapt comes back to your nervous system. If your nervous system is being challenged with the opportunity to recover, you will have better outcomes. If your exercise program is never varied or altered, your brain gets bored and conserves energy.

My fitness routine is 5 days per week. I workout first thing, starting sometime between 5 a.m. and 6 a.m. It's a time of day I won't be interrupted and I can give my first and best 10% of my day.

High-intensity, short-duration exercise formats

Here's a list of high-intensity, short-duration exercise formats that can help you build lean muscle and provide exercise variation.

Tabata. This is an exercise format done in intervals. For each exercise you spend 4 minutes alternating between 20 seconds of activity, as intensely as you can do it, followed by 10 seconds of rest. Tabata is the format I suggest you start doing on day 2 of *Your 7 Day Jump Start to Health*.

CrossFit. This is an exercise format that varies high-intensity functional movements by switching between exercises for strength, flexibility, balance, and seven other fitness areas. CrossFit is the format I follow and I do it at a gym (a.k.a. "box" in CrossFit lingo).

Could I do Crossfit, Tabata, or other lean-muscle-building exercises at home? Sure, but the "box" serves me both physically and socially, providing a community aspect that I can't get at home or in traditional gyms.

The point is that I found a format that works for me, making it easier to make sure I receive my movement nutrients in addition to a social connection and community. You need to do the same; find a format that works for you so you have movement sufficiency.

Can you pass the sitting-rising test?

Even if you are already a dedicated exerciser, do you really know how much good your fitness routine is doing for you? To find out, take the simple sitting-rising test (SRT), described in the European Journal of Preventive Cardiology (http://cpr.sagepub.com/content/early/2012/12/10/2047487312471759.abstract.

In the study, more than 2,000 adults ages 51 to 80, all part of an exercise program at Clinimex Exercise Medicine Clinic in Rio de Janeiro, took the sitting-rising test. People who scored fewer than eight points on the test were twice as likely to die within the next six years compared with those who scored higher; those who scored three or fewer points were more than five times as likely to die compared with those who scored more than eight points.

Overall, each point increase in the SRT score was associated with a 21% decrease in mortality from all causes.

A perfect score is 10. Do it for yourself. Maybe it will serve as a wake up call or a kick in the pants.

Test yourself

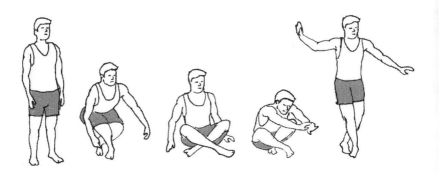

1. Stand in comfortable clothes in your bare feet, with clear space around you.

2. Without leaning on anything, lower yourself to a sitting position on the floor.

3. Now stand back up, trying not to use your hands, knees, forearms, or sides of your legs.

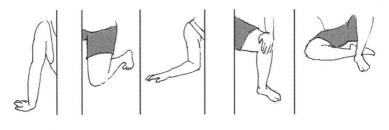

Hand: 1 point   Knee: 1 point   Forearm: 1 point   One hand on knee or thigh: 1 point   Side of leg: 1 point

Scoring

Use this chart to score how well you did.

		Points	
		Sitting	Rising
		5	5
1.	Subtract one point for each time you used any of the following for support: hand • knee • forearm • sides of legs *Example*: If you used two hands to sit, deduct two points.		
2.	Subtract 0.5 points if you lost your balance.		
3.	Subtotal your sitting and rising points.		
4.	Add your subtotals for a grand total.		

For a video on how to do the test, go to http://www.usatoday.com/story/news/2015/02/26/sitting-rising-test-life-expectancy-fitness/24076407/

Now that you know why movement is a nutrient, and inadequate movement leads to deficiency and toxicities in your body and your brain, this is a good place to move on to Part III, *Your 7 Day Jump Start to Health*. It gives you specific actions you can take in small steps to begin adding more sufficiency and purity to your health. It also gives you a good perspective of how I practice health and coach others to health. Our reward for pursuing health is having the physical, mental, chemical, and spiritual stamina needed to serve our families and fulfill our missions.

PART III

YOUR 7 DAY JUMP START TO HEALTH

In Part I, we unpacked the 4 Ps of steward leadership—philosophy, purpose, psychology, and procedures—by relating those concepts to taking care of your health.

In Part II, we covered the science of health from the perspective of the state that our bodies are in, protection and survival or growth and repair mode. We also learned about the five pillars that keep us in a cycle of illness, starting with chronic inflammation caused by food, busyness, and other lifestyle choices that stress our bodies.

In this part, we help you jump start your way to better health with a simple, 7 day plan. Here's the big picture:

Day	Jump Start
1	Drink and be glad.
2	Move different.
3	Find rest.
4	Supplement yourself.
5	Rule with raw.
6	Go pro.
7	Set a health goal.

Days 1-5 are meant to jump start your daily health routine, and days 6 and 7 to jump start your life-long health routine.

Here's how it works: Start with the steps on day 1. When you're comfortable you can do those steps, add the steps for day 2. When you're comfortable you can do both the day 1 and day 2 steps, and then move on to day 3. Repeat the routine for days 4 and 5 until you're doing the steps for days 1-5 on a daily basis.

The idea is to build on one day to the next. If you don't have the energy to move immediately from day 1 to day 2, and so on, then stay with day 1 until you feel up to day 2. If you need a week of day 1s then you need a week of day 1s. Depending on your biblical interpretation, the seven days can be literal or figurative. There's no wrong way to tackle this, except for not doing it at all. Now let's get started.

DAY 1: DRINK AND BE GLAD

Why jump start your health with drinking and gratitude? Because both can help calm your nervous system.

Day	Jump Start	Additive Actions
1	Drink and be glad.	• Drink pure water.
		• Be grateful to be glad.

If you have a chronic illness, then your nervous system is in constant protection and survival mode, and is out of balance. Adding pure water and gratitude are easy ways to urge your nervous system back to rest-and-digest growth mode.

To add water

1. If you don't already drink purified water, ask someone who does to fill a jug for you, or gather the coins to buy a gallon or more.

2. Use easy math—your body weight divided by 2—to find the target number of ounces you should consume daily, starting today.

3. Over the course of your day, drink your target number of ounces. For example, I weigh 160lbs so I try to drink 80 ounces of water—about two and half quarts—each day.

4. Eat a mineral-rich food or take a multi-*mineral* supplement to replenish your electrolytes.

5. Expect more bathroom breaks than usual.

Look at those steps again, and notice none of the steps involves giving up anything else you like to drink. If you just have to have your coffee or a beer today, that's fine, just make sure to drink a glass of water before you drink your other beverage. Also notice certain words in steps 1-4: target, purified, and electrolytes.

Strive to drink your target number of ounces, and don't fret if you don't quite get there. The key point is to drink more water than you already are.

Purified water includes distilled water, spring water, or reverse osmosis water (all plain, not carbonated). Whether you purify it yourself or buy it that way, be aware that some products or brands are better than others. For example, the purity of bottled water is limited by the processes the manufacturer uses to remove industrial or pharmaceutical pollutants. Purified water is *not* straight tap water, which is filled with industrial chemicals, hormones (from other people's pee), and pharmaceutical drugs.

Electrolytes are minerals that carry electrical charges such as sodium, calcium, potassium, and others. Your cells need electrolytes. The sheer quantity of water you drink could dilute your electrolytes and lead to more bathroom breaks. It's easy to replenish your electrolytes: you can eat a small snack of a mineral-rich food, such as bananas, citrus fruits, dark green vegetables, or nuts; drink a mineral rich liquid, such as chicken broth; take a multimineral supplement; or drink *spring* water. Spring water has minerals; other types of purified water do not. The price for purified water at health food stores ranges from 25 cents/gallon to refill your own jugs to $1/gallon (the price I pay for the convenience of bottled Eldorado spring water).

Notice I did not include commercial sports drinks as way

to restore electrolytes. Contrary to what the makers want you to believe, sports drinks do not improve your health, so avoid them. Remember the glycemic index chart in Chapter 9? Gatorade checked in at 78!

As for the bathroom breaks, be grateful because your body is filtering and flushing toxins as it (finally) should be.

To add gladness

1. Spend 25-60 seconds reflecting on what you are grateful for today.

2. Write it down and carry it with you today.

3. When life gets hectic today, or whenever you have a spare moment, pull it out and read it.

Gratitude is the best way to center yourself emotionally. What you are grateful for doesn't have to be profound or long. Simple and short is good enough. A list of one is okay.

Write what you are grateful for on something easy to carry, easy to find, and not too easy to lose. Perhaps write it on a sticky note, an index card, or the back of a bookmark. Then put it where it's always with you and you can quickly retrieve it, such as a pocket or purse, or taped to your cell phone. You could even write on first-aid tape and fasten it to your wrist.

When you're feeling frazzled or have a spare moment, use some speed to grab your gratitude reminder, but read it and speak it slowly. For example, each time you go to the bathroom, just whip out your little piece of paper of gratitude and read it. Be thankful you have a private toilet, indoor plumbing, and don't have to walk to an outhouse or dig a hole.

DAY 2: MOVE DIFFERENT

Study after study is calling sitting the new smoking. Inactivity is poison to the brain. Movement is *life*, internally and externally. You can consume the best nutrients on the planet but without movement, your body cannot use those nutrients.

So today you will repeat what you did on Day 1 plus you will start to move different by getting out of your chair.

Day	Jump Start	Additive Actions
1	Drink and be glad.	• Drink pure water.
		• Be grateful to be glad.
2	Move different.	• Stand and sit better.
		• Do some quick kick-butt exercise.

If the thought of doing anything more than writing down what you're thankful for and drinking 1/2 your body weight in ounces of water dismays you, then stop here; stay on Day 1 and be proud of what you've accomplished so far.

If you are ready for Day 2, then try to work in both standing and exercise. If at first you're only up to doing one or the other, that's ok, too.

To add standing and sitting

By "standing," I mean anything except traditional sitting. Here are some ideas on what you can use instead of a traditional chair:

• Sit on an exercise ball.

• Kneel on a cushion or yoga block.

- Elevate your work space and stand.

Before standing all day, every day, you may have to ease yourself into it. You can start by sitting on an exercise ball, with the next level kneeling on a cushion or yoga block. The more upright you are the better, and standing upright is better than sitting or kneeling. With all the water you're drinking, you'll be up pretty often anyway.

If you're wondering how to elevate your workspace, start with something easy and inexpensive like I did: a $100 closet organizer.

I've never used them, but for trendier and more expensive options you might consider an adjustable standing desk such as a VariDesk. Which leads us to your next jumpstart action: add easy, kick-butt exercise.

To add exercise

"Easy kick-butt" exercise means short-time—as little as 4 *minutes* per exercise—and *intense*. Now there's something to be thankful for: 4 minute exercises give you time for the bathroom from all that water you're drinking.

Why easy kick-butt and not, say, an hour on the treadmill? Answer: Short-time and high intensity gives you a big bang for your exercise buck because it's one of the best ways to build lean muscle tissue, regulate your insulin, balance your hormones, and feed your brain.

I like Tabata (after Dr. Tabata in Japan) exercise for a four-minute, four-step, high-intensity exercise format. To do it, you'll need:

- A timer or clock to track seconds. For an online timer and a smartphone app, try http://www.tabatatimer.com/

- A small area to move around in. A 6 ft x 6 ft area (a common distance between couch and TV) might be sufficient.

For each exercise you do, here are the steps:

1. Choose an exercise that promotes survival, such as situps, pushups, jumping jacks, pullups, or burpees. Or do something silly and fun with your kids. Dance around, do full body wiggles, or race them.

2. Do the exercise as intensely as you can for 20 seconds.

3. Rest for 10 seconds.

4. Repeat steps 2 and 3 for eight repetitions.

In step 1, I mentioned burpees. You get on the floor and stand up. It's a full body, no equipment, two-in-one strength and aerobic exercise, a.k.a. "squat thrust." Beginners can start by "walking it out." To find online instructions and videos, just search for "burpees."

Whatever exercise you do, hang in there for the entire four minutes if you can. It really makes a difference. If you can't do the whole routine right away, that's fine; push to add another 30 seconds the next time, moving from 2 minutes 30 seconds to 3 minutes and so on, until you work up to 4 minutes.

Eventually Day 2 will become second nature. You'll rarely be sitting and you'll be doing 4-12 minutes of Tabata or other short-time, high-intensity exercises each day. All that movement will help tire your body out so you'll be begging to go to bed and glad for a sleep routine.

DAY 3: FIND REST

By now, you should be spending most of your day on your feet and moving. A big part of movement is *knowing when to stop.*

Many leaders don't have a stopping problem because they're in a perpetual stop-sit-eat sugar-wheat-caffeine cycle. Consequently, they often sleep horribly. They've conserved so much energy and consumed so many stimulants through the day that by bedtime their bodies and brains are just getting revved up.

So today you'll add a routine to help yourself to well-earned quality sleep.

Day	Jump Start	Additive Actions
1	Drink and be glad.	• Drink pure water.
		• Be grateful to be glad.
2	Move different.	• Stand and sit better.
		• Do some quick kick-butt exercise.
3	Find rest.	• Create a sleep routine.

Your sleep routine involves preparing where you sleep for sleep, and going to bed at a regularly scheduled time. I know you'll have challenges like kids waking up, a pain keeping you up, a crappy mattress, or something else that's creating sleep dysfunction. Busyness in particular is a surefire way to impede sleep; so it's imperative that you break it before it breaks you.

In addition to helping you break busy, preparing your sleep space and sticking to a sleep routine helps balance your hormones, especially the growth hormone insulin. The better your body is in tune with insulin, the easier it is to lose weight, gain energy, and inhibit many disease processes like cancer. Control insulin, control your health. Sleep is one of the best ways to do that.

To find rest

Sleep is an activity that you need to prepare for just as you do for work, dinner, or your sermon. If you want quality sleep, then you need to have a routine that signals it's time for sleep. Here's how:

1. Move the TV to another room.

2. Move the kids to their rooms.

3. Move the pets to their kennels.

4. Put your cell phone out-of-sight and hearing.

5. Get rid of or cover *anything* that has a light.

6. Choose a regular bed time.

7. Every night—including weekends—be in bed within 30 minutes of your bed time.

Take a second look at the list: we take similar steps to prepare our kids for sleep, why not ourselves? The more regulated your sleep schedule, the less your nervous system is under stress; instead of guessing or being surprised by what's happening next; your nervous system knows what to expect. This gives it a chance to calm down, moving you from fight-or-flight protection mode to rest-and-digest growth mode.

DAY 4: SUPPLEMENT YOURSELF

I hope you are rested and at least planned out a rest schedule. Let's review and preview. First, look at what you've accomplished in three days and be proud! If you haven't done it all yet, no worries; just keep working on what doesn't overwhelm you, build on it when you're ready, and be thankful you are making progress.

Second, if you are ready to move on, then today you'll add supplements that contain the nutrients that your body really needs and probably isn't getting, no matter how diligent you are with food.

Day	Jump Start	Additive Actions
1	Drink and be glad.	• Drink pure water. • Be grateful to be glad.
2	Move different.	• Stand and sit better. • Do some quick kick-butt exercise.
3	Find rest.	• Create a sleep routine.
4	Supplement yourself.	• Add the supplements you *really* need. • Buy supplements with pure ingredients.

There are two questions I get on a daily basis about supplements: "Do I really need to supplements?" In a perfect world, like Eden, the answer is "No." But in highly industrialized America, the answer is "Yes." If you're not sure which world you live in, use this checklist to find out:

The Eden supplements-decision checklist

You do not need to take supplements if...

[ ] 1. You *only* eat local, organic, non-GMO, in season produce.

[ ] 2. You have *never* consumed antibiotics.

[ ] 3. You *only* eat wild game meat, fish, and fowl.

[ ] 4. You get 15-30 minutes of sun exposure *daily* and *naked*.

[ ] 5. You *only* drink pure, non-chemically treated water.

[ ] 6. You've *never* consumed alcohol, medications, or caffeine.

[ ] 7. You live in a world *before* 5,000 BC.

If you checked-in all of the boxes, then you live in an environment like the Garden of Eden. Otherwise, you need supplements. But how do you know what to take? On this matter, especially, I want you to do some critical thinking. You can devise your own test, or you can use mine.

To add the pure supplements you really need

The types of supplements you need depend on your nutrient deficiencies. The best way to know your deficiencies is by having lab work and analysis that goes beyond the "one size fits all" labs you may be getting during your routine checkup.

Having said that, there are four deficiencies that I have, my family has, I consistently see in my clients, and where supplements can help:

- cell building-block fats
- gut bacteria

- sunshine

- micronutrients

Now the conundrum is which supplements will give me the most bang for my buck? My test for any supplement has to pass three questions:

1. Is it a required nutrient for the body to function optimally?

2. Am I getting these regularly in my diet?

3. Is it pure? I don't want to supplement with something that I would never eat.

With that in mind, there are four supplements that I take and give to my family on a daily basis, and recommend to my clients.

Omega 3. This supplement has the fats that are the building blocks of virtually every cell in your body. Deficient cells are weak cells; they'll have a hard time regenerating, healing, and repairing. The best food sources of Omega 3 are wild game meat and truly fresh fish. I don't hunt or have access to hunted meat or truly fresh fish. Do you?

Probiotics. These are the bacteria that live in your gut. They affect 70% of your immune system and convert much of the food you eat into usable forms of nutrients like B vitamins. We are all deficient in these nutrients due to herbicides, pesticides, fungicides, radiation, and society's germa-phobe-antibacterial everything in our food and in our environment. I eat organic, but I'm also a good guest (not a social jerk). When I visit family or friends or attend social events, I eat what they eat.

Vitamin D. I covered vitamin D in detail in Chapter 12. Here's a recap of the key points: Your body uses vitamin D in over 2,000 genetic reactions; deficiencies contribute to ailments like MS, depression, cancers, obesity, and more; it's devilishly hard to get it from food, and only a bit easier to get it from the sun. I spend most of my days in my office, and the neighbors might be unhappy to have nude sunbathers in the 'hood. A vitamin D supplement clears the hurdles.

Juiced fruits and vegetables. Most of us (including me) find it challenging to shop for, prepare, and consume the sheer quantity of fresh fruits and vegetables needed to daily and adequately fuel our bodies. Drinking your produce makes it a little easier.

Buying the good, avoiding the bad

Walk into any grocery or drug store of any size, and you can easily be overwhelmed by the number of supplement brands they carry. Personally, I avoid the big-box stores; the brands they carry are cheaper for a reason.

Though a bit pricier than other brands, these are the ones I take because I'm confident they're made from pure ingredients:

- Innate Choice® EPA:DHA Omega 3

- Innate Choice® Probiotics

- Thorne Vitamin D

- Juice Plus+® as an easy alternative to liquid juicing

If you have any other questions about these or other supplements, just call or email to set up a free 15 minute phone consultation. You can find my contact information at http://www.morehealthlesshealthcare.com

DAY 5: RULE WITH RAW

Yesterday was pretty easy in just finding some supplements. You're probably wondering when I'm going to talk about food. Today is your lucky day. I promise to make it easy. I won't even take anything away.

Day	Jump Start	Additive Actions
1	Drink and be glad.	• Drink pure water.
		• Be grateful to be glad.
2	Move different.	• Stand and sit better.
		• Do some quick kick-butt exercise.
3	Find rest.	• Create a sleep routine.
4	Supplement yourself.	• Add the supplements you *really* need.
		• Buy supplements with pure ingredients.
5	Rule with raw.	• Eat raw fruit or vegetables first.
		• Eat non-fruit and non-vegetables second.

For some people, their biggest hurdle in adding raw produce is changing their beliefs about which types of foods taste better and are more satisfying: Is it the community-building staples containing sugar and wheat, or is it fresh fruits and vegetables? Knowing the raw rules can help with the mind switch.

To rule with raw

Rules can be "big truths" or guidelines for action, or—in the case of raw rules—both. Here are the rules:

The big truth. Eating raw fruits and vegetables helps your body build and maintain a healthy immune system and turns you into a cancer-fighting machine.

The rules for action. Eat some raw produce *before* eating any non-vegetable or non-fruit.

You don't have to give up breads, pastas, burgers, nachos, or German chocolate cake; just eat a salad, carrot, apple, or other produce first. Eventually, you'll naturally shift towards raw foods. That will happen because you'll be more aware of how much better you feel and function when you eat raw foods, and how poorly when you eat Frankenfood.

When you eat raw foods, you are singing a love song to your cells. Happy cells are healthy cells. Healthy cells lead you and your family to better health and less medical spending. Remember earlier, about spending wisely by aligning your health dollars with your 4 Ps.

DAY 6: GO PRO

Until now, you've been jump starting your health on a daily basis. If you're feeling a little overwhelmed with your additive improvements, then your anxiety level is likely proportional to the quantity and quality of change that your nervous system is trying to handle.

It's time for day 6 and adding something to your routine to help you attain life-long health.

Day	Jump Start	Additive Actions
1	Drink and be glad.	• Drink pure water.
		• Be grateful to be glad.
2	Move different.	• Stand and sit better.
		• Do some quick kick-butt exercise.
3	Find rest.	• Create a sleep routine.
4	Supplement your-self.	• Add the supplements you *really* need.
		• Buy supplements with pure ingredients.
5	Rule with raw.	• Eat raw fruit or vegetables first.
		• Eat non-fruit and non-vegetables second.
6	Go pro	• Get help from a Functional Chiropractor.

If your nervous system is overloaded from insufficiencies and toxicities, you may need outside help to recharge it. Think of it like your cell phone. You've been texting, updating Facebook, talking, web surfing, and playing Candy Crush and your battery is about dead. You need to plug it into an outlet to recharge it.

To go pro with your health

If it's your nervous system that needs recharging, then the "outlet" you want on your team is a *Functional* Chiropractor who, unlike other chiropractors, is someone who:

- Recognizes the body as an amazing healing, self regulating organism.

- Understands that the body doesn't work in parts; the body works as a system.

- Answers your nutrition questions from a purity and sufficiency paradigm.

- Advocates chiropractic as a tool in a healthy lifestyle, not as a checkbox in a hierarchy of medical services.

- Is comfortable helping people of any age towards health.

- Can analyze lab work.

- Shares your philosophy about what it means to be healthy.

I'm constantly gathering a network of health professionals who share my "More Health, Less HealthCare" vision. If you don't live in Colorado Springs, I'll do my best to help you find a Functional Chiropractor in your area. Just send an email to hello@drkurtperkins.com and include a few zip codes in your area. I'll get back to you with the name of someone I'd feel comfortable sending my family to. It doesn't have to be Colorado. I have connections all over the US and Canada.

DAY 7: SET A HEALTH GOAL

It's the final day of your 7-day jump-start, and the beginning of your steward leadership journey. It looks like this:

Day	Jump Start	Additive Actions
1	Drink and be glad.	• Drink pure water.
		• Be grateful to be glad.
2	Move different.	• Stand and sit better.
		• Do some quick kick-butt exercise.
3	Find rest.	• Create a sleep routine.
4	Supplement your-self.	• Add the supplements you *really* need.
		• Buy supplements with pure ingredients.
5	Rule with raw.	• Eat raw fruit or vegetables first.
		• Eat non-fruit and non-vegetables second.
6	Go pro.	• Get help from a Functional Chiropractor.
7	Set a health goal.	• Set a measurable health goal.
		• Have a great *why* for your goal.

God created the earth in six days and He's been working ever since. He's not part of the 4 Hour Week, set-it-and-forget-it system. As the steward of His creation, you need to be similarly diligent about your health. You've given your body a jump start; whatever your health goal is—to halt or reverse a chronic illness or something else—realistically, it may take 6, 12, or 24 months to achieve.

When I speak at events or work with clients, one of the

actions I push heavily is to set goals. Goals are not just wishes or dreams. Goals have achievable, objective *measures* as explained next.

To set a measurable health goal

When you set a goal, you *must* write it and keep it where you can see and read it every day. In your written goal include specifics about *why*, how much, by when, and how.

- For your why, use achievement-oriented words that help you define what you want but don't have.

- For your how much, make it countable so you can see progress.

- For your when, tie it to an event or passage of time that has meaning. You have to have an end date or you'll keep deferring it.

- For your how, be specific about the steps or methods you'll use. You need action steps so have a plan.

   Example of a weak goal. "I'll lose weight by eating more veggies and exercising every day."

   The goal lacks a why, lacks measures for how much and by when, and lacks steps.

   Example of a better goal. "I'll lose 20 pounds in 90 days. I'll accomplish it by eating greens, and doing Tabatas every day."

   Now the goal has some measures. Either you lost 20 pounds or you didn't; ate greens or you didn't; and so on. But it still lacks a why.

Example of a strong goal. "I'll weigh 175 pounds or less by Memorial Day so I can keep up with my kids on our hikes. I'll accomplish it by cutting out all sugar, eating greens with every meal, doing 20 minutes of Tabatas five days a week, and sleeping eight hours every night."

This is a goal! It has why, how much, when, and steps, making it easier to achieve and to mark progress while getting there. It also focuses on the positive end state (the weight you want to *be*).

The rest of your life

Now that you have a jump start on your health, then make choices every day that make you better, stronger, and faster. It all starts with your *why*, the core of your health goals and dreams. Having a great reason for your goal will motivate you to keep working on it when life gets rough. If you don't have a great *why*, you can get help from this book. Just go back to Part I and review the 4 Ps.

When it's time to make your next step, I pray for the Holy Spirit to nudge you and give you all the love and grace you deserve as you become a better steward of God's body so you can change the world the way He has called you.

In the meantime, remember health is an experience and journey that constantly takes work. Put the work clothes on and never take them off. You're going to do awesome.

Health is never owned. Health is merely rented and the rent is due every day.

Thanks Rory Vaden for letting me alter your quote, "Success is never owned, it's merely rented and the rent is due every day."

You, too, can substitute whatever noun you want into Rory's quote...health, leadership, maybe Steadership or Lewardship. You know what I mean.

Afterword

In the preface of this book, I wrote about growing up as a PK (preacher's kid) and coming to terms with the many illnesses and prayer requests for health that I witnessed among church members. Within the book, I also relate seeing my father's descent into Alzheimer's and my brother's early death; both situations that I believe were due to their servant-hostage leadership lives.

Here, I want to tell you a bit more about how my own childhood illnesses and advanced education led me to a calling as a functional chiropractor and why it's crucial for all Christians to take the mantle of steward leadership for our health.

As a child, I had chronic eczema, strep throat, bronchitis, and ear infections. I also remember that in addition to the prayer requests, many potlucks where church members had a Dixie Cup with colorful pills and capsules at their place setting. I thought these were candies and would get angry at the unfairness of why they got candy and I didn't, until I learned that those colorful things were medications.

As I matured, my own illnesses continued, and I noticed the prayer requests continued apace and the Dixie Cups were much fuller. My great internal debate was, "If God can heal why were we sick, and if medication is supposed to make us healthy, why weren't these people getting well?"

This dilemma set my career to a health-oriented one. If pills are meant to make us better and these people weren't getting better, then they must be getting the wrong pills. I had all the intentions of finding or developing the right medications so their prayers could be answered.

I came to a crossroads in my undergraduate biochemistry training concerning what created health. Was it DNA or environment? Was sickness caused by bad bugs, bad genes, or bad luck? Or was there something else to the equation?

One of my tasks as a lab assistant was to create petri dishes for cells to grow. I used the exact same cell lineage for every experiment, meaning the DNA was *always* the constant in the equation.

The "aha" moment was discovering that if I changed the petri dish environment, then the cells would have a different health expression. If the environment for one cell can affect health, why can't the environment of 70 trillion cells (you and me) change health expression? Drugs were an option to change the expression but it never got to the root cause of the problem. Medications are given to alter how the body communicates *after* an unfavorable outcome. Using medication is a reactive event.

What if instead of being reactive to a situation, I was able to help create a favorable environment in which the cell in the petri dish (or you and I) would flourish? This set the journey of *More Health, Less Healthcare*. Naturally, I experimented on my self and realized I was reversing my chronic eczema, bronchitis, and other illnesses. If it worked for me—someone with a family history of illness—why couldn't what I was doing for myself work for others? I mean, genetically, humans are more similar than tomatoes.

There had to be basic rules and foundations that allowed any human to express his or her full potential. The more I experimented and the more I experienced my own changes and witnessed changes with others, I *knew* that humans were predisposed to unbelievable health.

People in the church don't have to suffer. God already created an innate genetic intelligence to keep us healthy, strong, and vibrant. We just have to follow instructions and create a culture of stewardship to help our bodies THRIVE as God intended. Everyone has different life experiences that influence their health expression but no one is exempt from certain health principles.

And that's what this book has been about: providing you the tools, techniques, and strategies to start your physical stewardship journey. You deserve it. You're worth it. God expects it.

Has this book made a difference in your beliefs, thoughts, or behavior? Are you healthier now? I would love to hear about your journey and your success. Drop me a note at hello@drkurtperkins.com.

Thank You

Lindsay, my wife, for encouraging me to pursue my passion; for your steadfastness and energy in this game we call life; for being a rockstar wife and mom; and for being gentle and loving when my Ps don't align and steering me back on track.

Dr. Patrick Gentempo, for making philosophy cool and sexy; for guidance in identifying and clearing contradictions before destruction sets in; for influencing and being a mentor to so many in our profession; and for inspiring me to begin this book with the 4 Ps. "You never know how far-reaching something you may say or do today will affect the leaders of tomorrow."

Dr. James Chestnut, for being the ultimate example of living in alignment with a philosophy, purpose, psychology, and procedures; in short, an example that I can observe and be proud to share with my patients and family.

The Tuesday morning crew for always having my back, constant encouragement, and being excited for other's success.

John, Dave, Becky, and *Chad*, for honest feedback in this process.

Made in the USA
San Bernardino, CA
29 July 2018